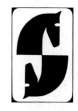

Cerebral Angiomas

Advances in Diagnosis and Therapy

Edited by
H. W. Pia J. R. W. Gleave E. Grote J. Zierski

With 161 Figures

Springer-Verlag
New York · Heidelberg · Berlin 1975

Symposium held in Gießen January 10–12, 1974 on the occasion of 20 years in Gießen

ISBN 0-387-07073-7 Springer-Verlag New York Heidelberg Berlin
ISBN 3-540-07073-7 Springer-Verlag Berlin Heidelberg New York

Library of Congress Cataloging in Publication Data. Main entry under title: Cerebral angiomas.
Papers presented at a meeting held Jan. 11–12, 1974 at Giessen. Bibliography: p. Includes index.
1. Brain--Tumors--Congresses. 2. Angioma--Congresses. I. Pia, Hans Werner, ed. [DNLM:
[DNLM: 1. Brain neoplasms--Congresses. 2. Hemangioma--Congresses. WL358' I58' 1974]
RC280.B7I56 616.9'92'81 74-28227
Printing and bookbinding: Offsetdruckerei Julius Beltz, KG, Hemsbach

Preface

The basic principles of the management of cerebral arteriovenous malformations were established during the first phase of the neurological attack on these problems between 1930 and 1960. The leaders were CUSHING, BAILEY and DANDY, but principally OLIVECRONA, and in Germany TÖNNIS. The experience gained showed that complete excision of the arteriovenous angioma was the only certain cure, and therefore was the procedure of choice.

In the present second phase important advances should be made and indeed are occurring. New diagnostic techniques such as total angiography, selective and superselective angiography, intraoperative and fluorescein angiography, and the EMI-scanner have been developed. The pathophysiological aspects have been further investigated by indirect and direct measurement of local and general cerebral blood flow.

Parallel with these developments operative technique itself has been improved and modified by new methods. A more aggressive attitude has been stimulated towards those angiomas, which had to be regarded as inoperable only a few years ago. Among these many improvements and technical advances include microsurgical techniques, combined stereotactic and microsurgical procedures, artificial embolization of different kinds and the cryosurgical management.

Multiple variables such as the age of the patient, the type, localization, and size of the angioma, its clinical picture and the possible complications, such as hemorrhage have been analysed and are understood better. These factors influence the indication for, and choice of, the appropriate procedure to a great extent.

The 20th anniversary of my work in Giessen, after 20 years of neurosurgery at Giessen University, has given the occasion for the discussion of the present position with regard to assessment and treatment of inoperable angiomas in a workshop together with experts in this field. The workshop, which was held Jan. 11.–12. 1974, was possible thanks to the generosity of Mr. and Mrs. H. KRÖNER of Fresenius Company, Bad Homburg.
This volume contains the papers and discussions of this meeting. The interest, which it aroused, led to rapid publication. The editors take great pleasure in expressing their thanks to the contributors for their participation and cooperation, and to Springer-Verlag for personal and technical aid in preparing and publishing the proceedings.

ipation and cooperation, and to Springer-Verlag for personal and technical aid in preparing and publishing the proceedings.
We hope that they may contribute to giving a more precise answer to the problem of how to deal with patients who suffer from the so-called inoperable cerebral angiomas.

Giessen, November 1974   HANS WERNER PIA

Contents

List of Editors and Contributors

AGNOLI, A. L.   Gießen, Zentrum für Neurochirurgie der Universität Gießen

BAUER, B. L.   Gießen, Zentrum für Neurochirurgie der Universität Gießen

BECK, B.   Bad Nauheim, W. G. Kerckhoff-Herzforschungsinstitut der Max-Planck-Gesellschaft

BEKS, J. W. F.   Groningen/Niederlande, Kliniek voor Neurochirurg., Academisch Ziekenhuis

BERGLEITER, R.   Stuttgart, Neuroradiologische Abteilung des Katharinenhospitals der Stadt Stuttgart

BRAUN, W.   Wuppertal-Elberfeld, Neurochirurgische Abteilung des Krankenhauses Bethesda

BURNEY, R. E.   APO New York 09220, USAF Hospital Box 582

BUSHE, K.-A.   Göttingen, Neurochirurgische Universitätsklinik

DJINDJIAN, R.   Paris/France, Département de Neuroradiologie Hôpital Lariboisière

ERBSLÖH, F.   Gießen, Zentrum für Neurologie der Universität Gießen

FEINDEL, W.   Montreal/Canada, Department of Neurology and Neurosurgery, McGill University and Montreal Neurological Hospital

GLEAVE, J. R. W.   Cambridge/Great Britain, Neurosurgical Department, Addenbrooke's Hospital

GROTE, E.   Gießen, Zentrum für Neurochirurgie am Klinikum der Justus-Liebig-Universität Gießen

HEKSTER, R. E. M.   Leiden/Niederlande, Neuroradiologische Abteilung, Academisch Ziekenhuis

HEMMER, R.   Freiburg i. Brsg., Neurochirurgische Universitätsklinik

JELLINGER, K.   Wien/Austria, Neurologisches Institut der Universität Wien

JOHNSON, R.   Manchester/Great Britain, Department of Neurological Surgery, Royal Infirmary

KOHLMEYER, K.   Gießen, Zentrum für Neurologie der Universität Gießen

KUHLENDAHL, H.   Düsseldorf, Neurochirurgische Universitätsklinik

KUNC, Z.   Prague/Czechoslovakia, Department of Neurosurgery, Charles University

LAPRAS, C.   Lyon/France, Hôpital Neurologique

LOEW, F.   Homburg, Neurochirurgische Universitätsklinik

LUESSENHOP, A. J.   Washington/U.S.A., Division of Neurological Surgery, Georgetown University Hospital

NADJMI, M.   Würzburg, Neuroradiologische Abteilung der Neurolog. u. Neurochirurg. Universitätskliniken

PAMPUS, F.   Stuttgart, Neurochirurgische Klinik des Katharinenhospitals der Stadt Stuttgart

PEETERS, F.   Nijmegen/Niederlande, Neuroradiologie – Neurochirurgische Abteilung des St. Radbond-Ziekenhuis und St. Canisius-Ziekenhuis der Universität Nijmegen

PENNING, L.   Groningen/Niederlande, Department of Neuroradiology, University Hospital

PENZHOLZ, H.   Heidelberg, Neurochirurgische Universitätsklinik

PERRET, G.   Iowa City/U.S.A., Division of Neurosurgery, University of Iowa Hospitals and Clinics

PIA, H. W.   Gießen, Zentrum für Neurochirurgie der Universität Gießen

RIECHERT, T.   Freiburg i. Brsg., Neurochirurgische Universitätsklinik

SANO, K.   Tokyo/Japan, Department of Neurosurgery, Univ. of Tokyo

SCHEPELMANN, F.   Gießen, Zentrum für Neurochirurgie der Universität Gießen

SCHÜRMANN, K.   Mainz, Neurochirurgische Universitätsklinik

SEEGER, W.   Gießen, Zentrum für Neurochirurgie der Universität Gießen

TZONOS, T.   Stuttgart. Neurochirurgische Klinik des Katharinenhospitals der Stadt Stuttgart

VOGELSANG, H.   Hannover, Abteilung für Neuroradiologie, Institut für klinische Radiologie der Medizinischen Hochschule Hannover

WALDER, H. A. D.   Nijmegen/Niederlande, Neurochirurgische Abteilung des St. Radbond-Ziekenhuis und St. Canisius-Ziekenhuis der Universität Nijmegen

WALTER, W.   Erlangen, Neurochirurgische Universitätsklinik

WÜLLENWEBER, R.   Bonn, Neurochirurgische Universitätsklinik

ZIERSKI, J.   Gießen, Zentrum für Neurochirurgie der Universität Gießen

The Indications and Contraindications for Treatment or Assessment

Introduction

H. W. PIA

It is believed that Fedor KRAUSE was one of the first neurosurgeons
to operate upon cerebral angiomas when in 1908 in Berlin he tried to
ligate the feeding vessels. However, the era of operative treatment
did not start until the thirties during which period CUSHING and BAI-
LEY reported 9 cases, DANDY 8 cases, and OLIVECRONA, TÖNNIS, and BERG-
STRAND published their classical monograph in 1936. They established
the principles of diagnosis and treatment: diagnosis based on the angiographic evaluation of the structure of the malformation, the number,
localization, and function of the feeding arterial vessels; and treatment based on the complete extirpation of the malformation where possible. Out of 20 intracranial arterio-venous angiomas 3 were totally
excised, the first by OLIVECRONA in 1932. In 2 cases the attempt had
to be abandoned, 4 cases were only explored, 3 patients had the intracranial arterial feeding vessels ligated; in 4 patients ligature of the
internal carotid artery was performed, and 3 patients were treated by
X-ray therapy.

Total excision was limited to small angiomas, in whom the occlusion
of the feeding vessels was possible before the draining veins were
approached. Angiomas situated in the motor area, the Sylvian fissure,
and the speech areas were considered inoperable. "The risk of rendering
a patient with seizures and perhaps only slight disturbance of function
hemiplegic and aphasic is not abolished by the technique of vessel ligation which is of doubtful value". The intracranial ligation of vessels was successful in only one case with a single feeding artery.

This pioneering work of OLIVECRONA and TÖNNIS is particularly impressive even on review of their results 20 years later. OLIVECRONA and
LADENHEIM reported in 1957 a series of 125 angiomas, out of which 81
were totally excised. 7 patients died, 50 were cured, 15 improved, and
7 became worse. TÖNNIS reported a series of 134 angiomas, out of which
56 were totally excised. 5 patients died. 61% of the survivors had full
working capacity, 22% were partially employed, and 11% were invalids.
Other large series from KRAYENBÜHL (15a) with 72 cases, MCKISSOCK and
HANKINSON (21) with 106 cases, NORLEN (23) with 57 cases, KRENCHEL (16)
with 98 cases, and FRENCH, CHOU and STORY (12) with 82 cases confirmed
such results.

OLIVECRONA summarized his experiences in 1957 with the following words:
"As matters stand today, if a patient with a lesion, which meets the
standards of operability undergoes extirpative surgery under hypotensive anesthesia, the likelihood of surgical mortality should be negli-
gible. About 85% of these patients will be clinically improved with

1

complete excision of the angiomatous tissue and freedom from future hemorrhage. Few of the remaining 15% will suffer any detriment.

1. The lesion may be totally removed, but the preexisting symptoms will be somewhat aggravated. This is a small premium to pay for insurance against further vascular accidents.

2. A small residue of angiomatous tissue may remain, but the symptoms will be improved.

3. Residual tissue may persist with aggravation of the preoperative symptoms. This last group may require further surgical intervention at a later date".

In spite of the overwhelming evidence of the effectiveness of extirpation of operable angiomas even in such cases many questions remain unsolved. This concerns particularly the prognosis of such important symptoms as epilepsy and hemorrhage which of course has a bearing on the question of the indications for surgery. Epileptic seizures were abolished in approximately 50% of patients (MCKISSOCK, TÖNNIS, NORLEN). In a few cases extirpative surgery led to epilepsy. Elimination of the danger of hemorrhage by total extirpation must be considered in relation to its prognosis which in spite of a recurrent hemorrhage rate between 40 and 60% is often quite good.

Palliative surgical procedures proved to be unsatisfactory. Out of 44 cases treated by OLIVECRONA 14 died, 2 following surgery, and 12 probably from later intracranial hemorrhage. 30 patients survived, 14 in good condition, but 9 were partial and 7 were complete invalids.

Afferent ligation, as performed by DANDY, should be considered only in cases where one single artery feeds the malformation, but even here the temptation should be resisted as arteriography is not infallible, and contributing vessels may not be demonstrated.

The electrocoagulation of surface vessels (TRUPP and SACHS) gave unsatisfactory results.

Carotid ligation should be given up. Not only was there no effect on the angioma, but the procedure was dangerous.

After ligation the blood flow through the angioma was derived from collateral sources, thus increasing, as we would say now, the steal effect. Radiation, as employed by CUSHING, was without the slightest discernible benefit. OLIVECRONA took a strong stand against the revival of this ineffectual form of therapy for arterio-venous malformations.

The indications for operation followed the rules of tumor surgery. Angiomas located in the functionally less important areas were considered to be surgically approachable. Small angiomas in the motor cortex were also removed; but in larger lesions the postoperative deficit constituted a greater handicap than the preoperative occassional seizure. Angiomas in the Sylvian fissure were often removed.

Intracerebral hemorrhage per se did not contraindicate prompt surgery when the condition of the patient might otherwise be endangered by delay, for the removal of the clot often exposes a partially mobilized lesion.

In angiomas in the region of the basal ganglia and internal capsule, in large malformations of the dominant hemisphere, and in most angio-

2

mas of the cerebellum and cerebello-pontine angle, surgery was contra-indicated. The same was true in cases of epilepsy of long standing, as there was little to gain from operation.

"In the absence of an absolute rule to guide his decision, the surgeon must carefully plot each borderline case against the abscissa of danger and the ordinate of benefit".

The last decade has brought important advances. The clinical symptomatology and course, and last but not least the natural history of unoperated cases has been studied and understood better, especially in the cooperative study by PERRET and NISHIOKA (26) and by WALTER (1970). Further progress was made by the introduction of preoperative total angiography and peroperative angiography, superselective angiography (DJINDJIAN), and magnification angiography. These investigations improved the diagnosis of small malformations and our knowledge of the pathomorphology of angiomas.

The pathophysiological aspects were advanced among others by SCHIEFER and TÖNNIS (39) and FEINDEL (9, 10) who elaborated upon the general and local cerebral blood flow disturbances. Current investigations by BECK and BAUER on the influence of the cerebral shunt on the heart and circulation may contribute to the better understanding of local and general compensation and decompensation mechanisms.

Parallel to these developments operative technique itself has been improved and this has stimulated a more aggressive attitude towards angiomas in functionally important areas. KUNC (18) reported on 97 angiomas out of which 58 were operated on; 7 were located in the speech area, 19 in the sensori-motor cortex, 5 in the Sylvian fissure, and 27 close to the above regions. Radical removal was possible in 48 cases with 8 deaths. On the other hand SANO, AIBA and JIMBO (36) stressed the high morbidity. In their series of 108 patients, 81 were operated upon. There was only one postoperative death, but 81% of patients had definite though variable residual neurological deficits.

The indications for radical removal of medial and paramedial angiomas are far from well defined and considerable reluctance is apparent. An important contribution was made by RIECHERT and MUNDINGER (35) who introduced a combined stereotactic and conventional procedure. The advantage of their method is the precise localization of the angioma with the possibility of an approach which causes the least functional disability. RIECHERT reported in 1972 16 cases of deep lying malformations on which successful operations have been carried out.

The use of the operating microscope was an undubitable and important step forward in the treatment of angiomas as was shown by RIECHERT and many others at the microsurgical symposia in Zürich (1968), Vienna (1972), and Kyoto (1973).

BUSHE (3) in a series of 42 cases treated 6 angiomas located in the midline, 7 in the ventricular and paraventricular region, and 2 in the basal ganglia. Radical removal was performed in 10 cases, vessel ligation in 2, and no operation in 3 cases. 2 patients died. DRAKE reported recently on 6 angiomas in the midbrain and pons, all successfully removed. The review of WALTER and BISCHOF (45) comprising 72 cases with angiomas located in those regions revealed that there were only 16 patients in whom the angioma was completely extirpated and 3 of them died. 16 further patients had partial ligation and out of this number 6 died.

Angiomas of the cerebellum were reported less frequently in earlier
series. Latterly VERBIEST (42), PIA (29), LAPRAS (1972) and YASARGIL
(46) and others have shown that even huge angiomas of this area have
become accessible due to improved technique especially the use of the
microscope.

Huge angiomas of the external and internal carotid system are regarded
as inoperable in most cases.

My own contributions to the emergency treatment of angiomas associated
with intracerebral and intraventricular hematomas (PIA 1968, 1972)
have shown that this can be a life-saving procedure with considerable
benefit also on morbidity. The operation risk is minimal, a contraindication exceptional.

It is to LUESSENHOP that the credit is due for introducing artificial
embolization in 1960 for the treatment of inoperable angiomas. He also
showed the effectiveness of such treatment. Incomplete embolization of
the angioma may facilitate or permit a total extirpation at a second
stage. SANO in 1965, and in Germany TZONOS, BERGLEITER and PAMPUS, as
well as SEEGER, have applied and modified the method of LUESSENHOP. A
further step forward was made by DJINDJIAN in 1970 who combined superselective angiography with embolization in a one stage procedure and
reported excellent results in arteriovenous malformations of the skull
and soft tissues of the face as well as in spinal angiomas. A glomus
tumor was successfully treated by embolization by HEKSTER, LUYENDIJK
and MATRICALI (13).

The freezing technique was developed by WALDER (1970) in order to throm-
bose the pathological vessels of inoperable and deep seated angiomas.
Cryosurgery may also be used as a complementary procedure after incomplete extirpation of a deep lying angioma.

X-ray therapy of arteriovenous angiomas is almost generally regarded
as ineffective. However, in 1955 POTTER reported on 10 patients treated by X-ray therapy out of which one died and 9 survived, 4 of them
for more than 20 years.

The similar experience of JOHNSON (14) suggests that X-ray therapy may
exert a favourable effect at least upon some forms of arteriovenous
malformations, so that we may have to reconsider the indications for
X-ray therapy in selected inoperable cases.

The basic principles of management of cerebral arteriovenous malformations were laid down during the first phase of therapy between 1932
and the mid-sixties. Experience showed that complete excision of the
angioma was the only method of cure, and therefore was the procedure
of choice.

In the present second phase not only have new techniques been developed
but also multiple variables such as the age of the patient, the type,
location, and size of the angioma; its influence on the cerebral and
general circulation, the clinical picture and possible complications,
such as hemorrhage and deficits produced by surgery, were analysed and
understood better. These factors influence the indication for and choice
of the appropriate procedure to a great extent.

The subject of this workshop is the treatment of inoperable angiomas.
I think that starting from this borderline position, we should try to
define the principles of management of patients with such lesions. I
hope also that we will try to define objective criteria for the choice

of treatment of different types of angiomas in general. The participation of so many distinguished experts from different specialties
makes me confident that we will come closer to our aim of answering
more precisely the question of how to deal with those patients who
have so-called "inoperable angiomas".

R e f e r e n c e s

1. BERGSTRAND, H., OLIVECRONA, H., TÖNNIS, W.: Gefäßmißbildungen und
    Gefäßgeschwülste des Gehirns. pp. 181. Leipzig: Georg Thieme 1936.

2. BROOKS, B.: The treatment of traumatic arterio-venous fistula.
    Sth. med. J. (Birmingham) 23, 100-106 (1930).

3. BUSHE, K. A., PETERSON, E., SCHÄFER, E. R.: Surgical Indication
    for Arteriovenous Angiomas in Functionally Important Regions and
    in Case of Spreading within the Area of the Ventricular System
    and of the Basal Ganglia. In Present Limits of Neurosurgery, Avi-
    cenum, Czechoslov. Med. Press, 299-302. Prague 1972.

4. CUSHING, H., BAILEY, P.: Tumors arising from the blood vessels of
    the brain. Baltimore: C. C. Thomas 1928.

5. DANDY, W. E.: Arteriovenous aneurysms of the brain. Arch. Surg.
    17, 190-243 (1928).

6. DJINDJIAN, R., COPHIGNON, J., THERON, J., MERLAND, J. J., HOUDART, R.:
    L'embolisation en neuroradiologie vasculaire. Technique et indi-
    cations à propos de 30 cas. Nouv. Presse mèd. 33, 2153-2158 (1972).

7. DJINDJIAN, R., HOUDART, R., COPHIGNON, J.: Premiers essais d'em-
    bolisation par voie fémorale de fragments de muscle dans un cas
    d'angiome médullaire et dans un cas d'angiome alimenté par la
    carotide externe. Rev. Neurol. 125, 119-130 (1971).

8. DJINDJIAN, R., MERLAND, J. J., REY, A., THUREL, J., HOUDART, R.:
    Artériographie super-sélective de la carotide externe. Neuro-
    Chirurgie Paris 19, 165-171 (1973).

9. FEINDEL, W., GARRETSON, H., YAMAMOTO, Y. L., PEROT, P., RUMIN, N.:
    Blodd flow patterns in the cerebral vessels and cortex in man
    studied by intracarotid injection of radioisotopes and Coomassie
    Blue dye. J. Neurosurg. 23, 12-22 (1965).

10. FEINDEL, W., HODGE, Ch. P., YAMAMOTO, Y. L.: Epicerebral angio-
    graphy by Fluorescin during craniotomy. In Progr. Brain Research
    30, 471-477. Amsterdam-London-New York: Elsevier 1968.

11. FRENCH, L. A., CHOU, S. N.: Conventional Methods of Treating In-
    tracranial Arteriovenous Malformations. Progr. Neurosurg. 3, 275-
    361. Basel-New York: S. Karger 1969.

12. FRENCH, L. A., CHOU, S. N., STORY, J. L.: Cerebrovascular malfor-
    mations. Clinical Neurosurg., Vol. XI, Chapter 14. Baltimore:
    Williams and Wilkins Co. 1964.

13. HEKSTER, R. E. M., LEUYENDIJK, W., MATRICALI, B.: Transfemoral
    Catheter Embolization: A Method of Treatment of Glomus Jugulare
    Tumors. Neuroradiology 5, 208-214 (1973).

14. JOHNSON, R. T.: Surgery of Cerebral Hemorrhage. In Recent Advances in Neurology, 124-126. (Eds. Lord Brain and Maria Wilkinson). London: Churchill 1969.

15. KRAUSE, F.: Krankenvorstellung aus der Hirnchirurgie (Fall 4. Ang. venosum racemosum). Zbl. Chir. 35, 61-63 (1908).

15a. KRAYENBÜHL, H.: Discussion des rapports sur les angiomas supra-tentoriels. 1. Congr. Internat. de Neurochirurgie, 263-267. Bruxelles 1957.

16. KRENCHEL, N. J.: Intracranial racemose angiomas, a clinical study. Universitetsforlaget I. Aarhus (1961).

17. KUNC, Z.: Operability of Arteriovenous Malformations in Functionally Important Cortical Regions. In Present Limits of Neurosurgery, Avicenum, Czechoslov. Med. Press, 293-298. Prague 1972.

18. KUNC, Z.: Possibility of surgery in arteriovenous malformations in the anatomically important and dangerous regions of the brain. J. Neurol. Neurosurg. Psychiat. 28, 183 (1965).

18a. LAPRAS, C., TUSINI, G., THIERRY, A.: A propos de 8 observations cliniques d'angiomes de la fosse cérébrale postérieure. Congrès Soc. Neurochirurgie langue Franc. Lyon 1963.

19. LUESSENHOP, A.: Artificial Embolization for Cerebral Arteriovenous Malformations. Progr. neurol. Surg. 3, 320-362. Basel-New York: Karger 1969.

20. LUESSENHOP, A. J., SPENCE, W. T.: Artificial embolization of cerebral arteries. Report of use in a case of arteriovenous malformation. J. amer. med. Ass. 172, 1153-1155 (1960).

21. MCKISSOCK, W., HANKINSON, J.: The surgical treatment of the supratentorial angiomas. Rapports et discussions. 1er Congrès International de Neurochirurgie, Bruxelles 1957.

22. NORLÉN, G.: Arteriovenous aneurysms of the brain: Report of ten cases of total removal of the lesion. J. Neurosurg. 6, 475-494 (1949).

23. NORLÉN, G.: Die chirurgische Behandlung intracranieller Gefäßmißbildungen. A. Angiome. Handbuch der Neurochirurgie. Hrsg. H. Olivecrona und W. Tönnis, Bd. 4/II, S. 147-206. Berlin-Heidelberg-New York: Springer 1966.

24. OLIVECRONA, H., LADENHEIM, J.: Congenital arteriovenous aneurysms of the carotid and vertebral arterial systems. Berlin: Springer 1957.

25. OLIVECRONA, H., RIIVES, J.: Arteriovenous aneurysms of the brain: their diagnosis and treatment. Arch. Neurol. Psychiat. 59, 567-602 (1948).

26. PERRET, G., NISHIOKA, H.: Arteriovenous malformations. An analysis of 545 cases of cranio-cerebral arteriovenous malformations and fistulae reported to the cooperative study. J. Neurosurg. 25, 467-490 (1966).

27. PIA, H. W.: The Diagnosis and Treatment of Intraventricular haemorrhages. Progr. in Brain Research 30, 463-470 (1968).

28. PIA, H. W.: Diagnose und Therapie der Hirnblutungen im Kindesalter. Tijdschr. Geneesk. 24, 765-770 (1968) und Beiträge Neurochir. 15, 245-251 (1969).

29. PIA, H. W.: Vasculäre Mißbildungen und Erkrankungen der hinteren Schädelgrube und ihre Behandlung. HNO 17, 165-171 (1969).

30. PIA, H. W.: The Operative Treatment of Intracerebral and Intraventricular Hematomas. Acta Neurochir. 27, 149-164 (1972).

31. PIA, H. W.: The Surgical Treatment of Intracerebral Hematomas. In Present Limits of Neurosurgery, Avicenum, Czechoslov. Med. Press, 323-328. Prague 1972.

32. POOL, J. L.: Treatment of arteriovenous malformations of the cerebral hemisphere. J. Neurosurg. 19, 136-141 (1962).

33. POTTER, J. M.: Angiomatous malformations of the brain: their nature and prognosis. Ann. roy. Coll. Surg. (Engl.) 16, 227-243 (1955).

34. RIECHERT, T.: Die operative Versorgung von Blutungen im Bereich der Stammganglien. Therapiewoche 22, 1152-1153 (1972).

35. RIECHERT, T., MUNDINGER, F.: Combined stereotaxic operation for treatment of deep seated angiomas and aneurysms. J. Neurosurg. 21, 358-363 (1964).

36. SANO, K., AIBA, T., JIMBO, M.: Surgical treatment of cerebral aneurysms and arteriovenous malformations. Neurologia med.-chir. 7, 128-131 (1965).

37. TÖNNIS, W.: Symptomatologie und Klinik der supratentoriellen arteriovenösen Angiome. 1. Congr. Int. de Neurochirurgie. Les Editions Acta Med., 205-215. Belgica 1957.

38. TÖNNIS, W., SCHIEFER, W., WALTER, W.: Signs and symptoms of supratentorial arteriovenous aneurysms. J. Neurosurg. 15, 471-480 (1958).

39. TÖNNIS, W., SCHIEFER, W.: Zirkulationsstörungen des Gehirns im Serienangiogramm. Berlin-Göttingen-Heidelberg: Springer 1959.

40. TÖNNIS, W., WALTER, W.: Die Indikation zur Totalextirpation der intracraniellen arteriovenösen Angiome. Dtsch. Z. Nervenheilk. 186, 279-298 (1964).

41. TRUPP, M., SACHS, E.: Vascular tumors of the brain and spinal cord and their treatment. J. Neurosurg. 5, 354-371 (1948).

42. VERBIEST, H.: Arteriovenous aneurysms of the posterior fossa. In Progr. Brain Research 30, 383-396. Amsterdam-London-New York: Elsevier 1968.

43. WALDER, HAD.: Die Behandlung arteriovenöser Anomalien im Gehirn mit Hilfe von Kryotherapie. Therapiewoche 22, 1542-1543 (1972).

44. WALDER, HAD.: Freezing Arteriovenous Anomalies in Brain. In Avicenum, Czechoslov. Med. Press, 303-308. Prague 1972.

45. WALTER, W., BISCHOF, W.: Klinik und operative Behandlung der arteriovenösen Angiome des Stammhirns, bzw. der sogenannten Mittelhirnangiome. Neurochirurgie, $\underline{9}$, 150-166. Stuttgart 1966.

46. YASARGIL, G.: Report J. Int. mp. Microneurosurgery. Kyoto 1973.

Chapter I
Morphological Aspects

The Morphology of Centrally-situated Angiomas

K. JELLINGER

Angiomas are localized collections of blood vessels, abnormal in structure and in number, and composed of normal or malformed arteries, veins,
capillaries, or a mixture of these. Within the CNS, vascular malformations are usually congenital in origin and caused by faulty embryologic
development. They represent persistence of a primitive pattern of vascular pathways with anomalous structures and altered hemodynamics. Though
not true neoplasms, these vascular hamartomas may grow and inflict acute
or progressive damage on the brain tissue.

I n c i d e n c e

The rarity of these vascular lesions suggested by COURVILLE (3) is neither confirmed by clinical experience nor by personal figures from two
autopsy series in a University Medical Center and a Regional Neuro-Psy-
chiatric Center, where CNS angiomas were found in 0.35 and 0.87% of the
cases respectively (Table 1).

Table 1. Incidence of cerebral vascular malformations (CVM)

COURVILLE (1945):	30000 autopsies –	29 CVM (= 0.1 %)
	(1100 cerebral	18 telangiectasias
	hemorrhages)	5 venous angiomas
		5 venous varices
		1 AV angioma
Institute of Path.	5553 autopsies –	20 CVM (= 0.35 %)
Univ. of Vienna	(166 cerebral	6 telangiectasias
(1969-1971)	hemorrhages)	1 cavernous angioma
		1 venous angioma
		12 AV angiomas
Neuro-Psychiatr.	1600 autopsies –	14 CVM (= 0.87 %)
Hospital Linz	(43 cerebral	3 telangiectasias
(1968-1972)	hemorrhages)	2 cavernous angiomas
		3 venous angiomas
		6 AV angiomas

In neurosurgical material the incidence of cerebral angiomas varies from 0.5 - 7% and was 3.5% of the brain tumors confirmed by biopsy 1964-1972 at the Dept. of Neurosurgery, Univ. of Vienna, and 5% of the total of brain tumors in the files of the Neurological Institute Vienna. Vascular malformations are responsible for 10 - 40% of surgically treated intracranial hemorrhages (11) and for 1 - 5% of cerebral hematomas found at autopsy (5).

C l a s s i f i c a t i o n

Several types of vascular malformations in the CNS have been described. They have been classified 1. by size: a) small ("cryptic") angiomas (less than 2 cm in diameter), b) medium-sized (2-4 cm), and c) large angiomas (over 4 cm); 2. according to the location: a) supra- and in-fratentorial; b) superficial: cortical, subcortical; c) paramedial: basal ganglia and ventricles; d) medial: corpus callosum and brainstem; e) solitary, multiple and diffuse; and 3. by morphological appearance, a simple scheme distinguishing: a) capillary telangiectasias, b) cavernous angiomas, c) arteriovenous malformations, d) venous angiomas including varix formation. For review of the various malformations and of the distinguishing anatomical features of each of these types (7, 11).

Table 2. Morphological type of angiomas by location

a) McCORMICK et al. (7)

Type	Cerebral (n=346)	Cerebellum (n = 164)	Brainstem	Total
AV Angioma	217	52	18	287
Cavernous	59	11	10	80
Venous	46	20	11	77
Telangiect.	22	6	32	60
Varix	2	2	2	6

b) Personal series: 117 autopsies and 83 biopsies ( )

Type (+mult. 8)	Cerebral Hemisph.	Choroid Plexus	Basal Ganglia	Cerebellum	Brain Stem	Total
AV Angioma	33+(73)	4 (2)	12+(1)	4 (2)	12	56(78)
Cavernous	4+ (3)	-	1+	-	2	7 (3)
Venous	10	2 (1)	-	3	4	19 (1)
Telangiect.	5+ (1)	-	1	5	15	26 (1)
Total	52 (77)	6 (3)	14 (1)	12 (2)	33	117(83)

Table 2 compares the morphological type and location of cerebral angiomas in the series reported by McCORMICK et al. (7) and in a personal material of 200 cases (117 autopsies and 83 biopsies).

Morphological Types

a) <u>Telangiectasias</u> are small, mostly solitary groups of abnormally dilated capillaries separated by normal neural tissue. They are usually found incidentally at necropsy. Unlike other small or "cryptic" angiomas, they are most uncommonly associated with spontaneous hemorrhage. The most common site is the pons, less often the cerebellum and cerebral hemispheres are involved.

b) <u>Cavernomas</u> are composed of closely clustered, sinusoidal thin-walled vessels with no intervening nervous tissue. They range in size from pinpoint lesions to foci of several cm in diameter. They may be multiple and have been found in all parts of the CNS including the brain stem where they may cause fatal hemorrhage. Neither of these types of lesion have extra development of the vessels of supply which is typical for the next two types.

c) <u>Arteriovenous (AV) angiomas</u> constitute the most frequent vascular malformations of the CNS with greatly dilated and thickened vessels. There are irregular vascular cavities formed by arteries and veins of all sizes closely clustered and replacing the intervening and adjacent nervous tissue. Their size ranges from small examples to extensive tortuous masses occupying large parts of the brain. They occur in all parts of the CNS, but the larger ones most often involve the area supplied by the middle cerebral artery (6). Previously regarded as rare in other locations, almost 25% of all AV malformations are found in the posterior fossa (Table 2). Secondary degeneration, with fibrosis, venous dilatation, calcification, thrombosis with organisation, and evidence of old or recent hemorrhages, is frequently found. A rare variety in infancy and childhood is a dilatation or varix of the great vein of Galen which is often associated with obstructive hydrocephalus and congenital cardiac defects (9).

d) <u>Venous angiomas</u> are composed entirely of veins with one or more large draining veins. As in AV malformations, but unlike cavernomas, nervous parenchyma is found (Fig. 10). They occur in all parts of the CNS but are considered to be less common in the brain than in the spinal cord.

e) In small "<u>cryptic</u>" vascular malformations ("microangiomas") which are undetected by clinical investigations the gross appearance is unrewarding. The disclosure of these small lesions which include all morphological types, though chiefly AV angiomas, is dependent on careful microscopic examination. They have been found in all parts of the CNS.

Major Sites and Associated Lesions

With regard to treatment the morphologiacal classification of cerebral angiomas is of minor importance. The ideal treatment of a vascular malformation in the brain is radical excision, provided that the lesion is surgically accessible, and the risk of neurological deficit following surgery is minimal. Hence, the choice of treatment chiefly depends on the location and extent of the lesion and its vascular supply. Table 3 summarizes the major sites of cerebral angiomas, mainly AV mal-

Table 3. Percentage location of cerebral angiomas

Location	PERRET-NISHIOKA (10) 453 cases	BERRY et al. (1) 527 cases	KRAYENBÜHL & YASARGIL (6) 186 cases	MORELLO & BORGHI (8) 154 cases	McCORMICK et al. (7) 510 autopsies	Personal series 117 aut. 83 biop.
Cerebral hemispheres	80	85	75.1	80.1	(70	65
Corp. callos.		5	1.5			
Choroid plexus					(	4.5
Basal ganglia	2)	5)	8	7.7)		7.5)
Brainstem	)7	)10	2.6) 20.2	7.0) 19.9	13) 30	16) 35
Cerebellum	5	5	9.6	5.2	17	7
Diffuse/ Multiple	2		3.2			(4.0)
Not given	11					

formations, in several retrospective series (1, 6, 7, 8, 10). 65 -85%
of the angiomas involve the cerebral hemispheres, while up to 35% occur in the central parts of the brain. These deeply situated vascular
malformations will be discussed with reference to the therapeutic problems involved.

a) Cerebral Hemispheres: Many AV malformations are visible on the surface whence they extend as a wedge of abnormal vessels into the subcortical white matter with the apex directed toward the ventricles
(Fig. 5). Most supratentorial angiomas are supplied by the middle cerebral artery, although a dual or multiple supply may be demonstrated.
The superficial lesions are drained by passively enlarged cortical
veins, and the centrally located ones by the vein of Galen via the internal cerebral veins. Thrombosis of large vessels with organization
(Fig. 1) and hemorrhage is frequently found. Multiplicity is more common in cavernomas than in AV angiomas, although this latter type may
be located at various sites in both hemispheres and within the brainstem (Fig. 6).

b) Basal Ganglia and Ventricles: A considerable proportion of angiomas
lies deep within the brain substance, such as those in the basal ganglia
and periventricular region which may protrude into the ventricles (Fig.
2). In various retrospective series, lesions in these central areas
constituted 8 - 12% of all angiomas (Table 3), while SAHS et al. (12)
discovered intra- and periventricular lesions in 18% of all vascular
malformations. Centrally located angiomas arise from branches of the
choroidal and posterior cerebral arteries or are supplied by both the
middle cerebral and basilar arteries. Some lesions are limited to the
lenticular nuclei, thalamus or periventricular region, while others
involve large central parts of both hemispheres and extend into the basal
cisterns, chiasm and brainstem. A large AV angioma in the right thalamus and subthalamus was found in a 60 year-old man with over 30 years'
history of hemiballisms which had ceased after a final stroke with destruction of the oral-ventral thalamus, a sort of spontaneous stereotaxic treatment. Hemorrhage into the basal ganglia and lateral ventricle
is to be expected in most of these large angiomas (Fig. 2), but has also
been found to arise from "cryptic" malformations in the basal ganglia.
Autopsy of a 70 year-old female displayed a small AV malformation in
the thalamus as the cause of apoplexy.

Vascular malformations of the choroid plexus have been reported as another source of intraventricular hemorrhage in both neonates and adults
(2, 4, 11). These cryptic angiomas are unilateral and may involve all
parts of the ventricular system. Some of them are only revealed by mi-
croscopical examination. This type of lesion was seen in 5.2% of our
autopsy series and in 3.6% of the biopsy cases of cerebral angiomas.
6 were AV malformations and 3 were considered to be venous angiomas.
The age of the patients ranged from 7 weeks to 50 years. 5 such angiomas were associated with intraventricular hemorrhage rupturing into
the cerebral substance, the others were asymptomatic. In a 50 year-old
man with a fatal parietal hemorrhage, a cryptic AV angioma was noted
in the adjacent choroid plexus of the lateral ventricle (Fig. 13). Another AV malformation was excised from the lateral ventricle of a boy
aged 11 years with acute intracranial hemorrhage (Fig. 14), while a
cluster of abnormal veins with extremely thin walls was excised from
the lateral ventricle of a girl aged 7 weeks with hydrocephalus (Fig.
15). It is suggested that more instances of intraventricular angiomas
will be found in both early and adult life if the choroid plexus is
routinely examined.

c) Midbrain: Vascular malformations are often limited to or chiefly
situated within the mesencephalic tectum or may rostrally extend to

13

the thalamus. Mechanical obstruction of the aqueduct results in intermittent or sustained hydrocephalus (Figs. 3, 4). While AV malformations
are readily diagnosed by angiography, cavernomas without special vessels of supply may escape recognition, e.g. in a 27 year-old man with
occlusive hydrocephalus who died after a CSF shunting procedure from
acute hemorrhage into a large cavernoma of the midbrain. The early compression of the aqueduct is one of the principle reasons for the onset
of clinical symptoms in midbrain angiomas. Autopsy of a 75 year-old
woman with a 50 years' history of chronic headache, periodic vomiting,
nystagmus and oculomotor disturbances displayed an AV malformation of
the quadrigeminal plate.

A rare form of angioma of the midbrain is associated with homolateral
angiomatosis of the retina and a trigeminal cutaneous nevus. This "mes-
encephalo-oculo-facial angiomatosis" (14) was seen in a 14 year-old
girl who died after proximal carotid occlusion. The cause of death
due to vascular malformation within the mesencephalon is usually massive hemorrhage (Fig. 4).

A variety of AV malformation consists largely of an impressive dilatation or varix of the great vein of Galen which may cause compression
of the brainstem and aqueduct. Basal angiodysgenesia with formation of
AV shunts between the basal cerebral arteries and the vein of Galen is
often associated with congenital cardiac defects, hydrocephalus and
cystic destruction of the brain (Fig. 12). The ultimate prognosis of
this rare lesion is poor.

d) Pons and Medulla: The most common type of angioma of the lower
brainstem is a clinically silent telangiectasis, although other vascular malformations do occur in the pons and medulla. The arterial component is invariably traced to the vertebral and basilar arteries;
drainage is accomplished through the veins of Galen and Rosenthal.
A large number of angiomas of appreciable dimensions involving the pons
were almost free of symptoms (Fig. 8). The reasons for the late appearance of clinical signs in brainstem angiomas are not clear. Massive
hemorrhage arising from AV and venous malformations may be limited to
the brainstem (Figs. 9, 10) or enters the fourth ventricle and is frequently the terminal event. A venous malformation was found as the
source of pontine bleeding in a 13 year-old boy who died after correction of Fallot's tetralogy.

e) The Cerebellum is more frequently affected by angiomas than the
brainstem (Table 3) but was the least often involved site in our series.
The deep angiomas within the lateral cerebellar white matter tend to be
small and of little clinical significance. The midline surface malformations within the vermis and subjacent to the tentorium are the largest. The brachium conjunctivum and neighboring pontine tegmentum are
frequently incorporated into the vascular mass (Fig. 7). The arterial
contributions stem from the terminal branches of the superior cerebellar artery. Although hydrocephalus may result from angiomas in the
vermis, the disturbances associated with cerebellar angiomas are not
distinguished by a prolonged course. This is illustrated by the case
of a 12 year-old girl without a history of neurological abnormalities
who expired within a few hours from a large cerebellar hemorrhage from
a ruptured AV angioma (Fig. 11).

S u m m a r y

Vascular malformations of the CNS can be morphologically classified as 1. capillary telangiectasias, 2. cavernomas, 3. arteriovenous malformations (including varix of the great vein of Galen), and 4. venous angiomas. A review of 200 personal observations (117 autopsies and 83 biopsies) and of various retrospective series indicates that about 35% of cerebral angiomas occur in central regions of the brain, i.e. the deep hemispheral white matter, the ventricles and periventricular areas (choroid plexus!), the basal ganglia, brainstem, and cerebellum. The major types of vascular malformations seen in the deep cerebral regions are described with reference to their anatomical features, their chief arterial supply and venous drainage, and their most frequent complications.

R e f e r e n c e s

1. BERRY, R. G., ALPERS, B. S., WHITE, J. C.: Angiomas. In: Cerebrovascular disease. C. H. Millikan, ed. Baltimore: Williams and Wilkins 1966.

2. BUTLER, A. B., PARTAIN, R. A., NETSKY, M. G.: Primary intraventricular hemorrhage. Neurology (Minneap.) 22, 675-687 (1972).

3. COURVILLE, C. B.: Pathology of the nervous system, 2nd ed. Mountina View, Cal.: Pacific Press Publ. Ass. 1945.

4. DOE, F. D., SHUANGSHOTI, S., NETSKY, M. G.: Cryptic angioma of the choroid plexus. Neurology (Minneap.) 22, 1232-1239 (1972).

5. JELLINGER, K.: Zur Ätiologie und Pathogenese der spontanen intrazerebralen Blutung. Therapiewoche 22, 1440-1449 (1972).

6. KRAYENBÜHL, H., YASARGIL, M. G.: Klinik der Gefäßmißbildungen und Gefäßfisteln. In: H. Gänshirt, ed., Der Hirnkreislauf, pp. 465-511. Stuttgart: G. Thieme 1972.

7. McCORMICK, W. F., HARDMAN, J. M., BOULTER, T. R.: Vascular malformations ("angiomas") of the brain, with special reference to those occurring in the posterior fossa. J. Neurosurg. 28, 241-251 (1968).

8. MORELLO, G., BORGHI, G.P.: Cerebral angiomas. Acta neurochir. (Wien) 28, 135-155 (1973).

9. NOETZEL, H., ZORGER, B.: Angiodysplasie der basalen Hirnarterien mit Varix der Vena magna Galeni. Z. Kinderchir. 5, 156-166 (1967).

10. PERRET, G., NISHIOKA, H.: Cerebral angiography. J. Neurosurg. 25, 98-116, 467-490 (1966).

11. PIA, H. W.: The surgical treatment of intracerebral and intraventricular haemoatomas. Acta neurochir. 27, 149-164 (1972).

12. RUSSELL, D. S., RUBINSTEIN, L. J.: Pathology of tumours of the nervous system, 3rd ed., pp. 91-108. London: Arnold 1971.

13. SAHS, A. L., PERRET, G. E., LOCKSLEY, H. B.: Intracranial aneurysms and subarachnoid hemorrhage. A cooperative study . Philadelphia: J. B. Lippincott 1969.

14. WYBURN-Masson, R.: Arteriovenous aneurysms of midbrain and retina, facial naevi and mental changes. Brain <u>66</u>, 163-203 (1943).

Table I (Legends see p. 17)

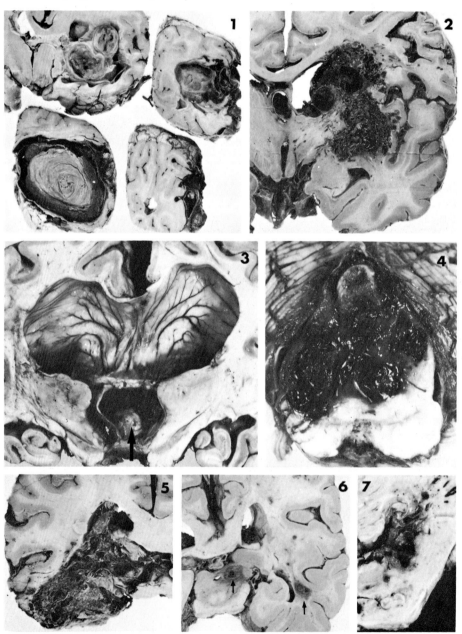

Table I

Fig. 1. Giant AV malformation in deep temporo-occipital white matter with extensive thrombosis in 23-year-old female

Fig. 2. Deep AV angioma in basal ganglia with recent hemorrhage in 30-year-old male

Figs. 3, 4. Obstructive hydrocephalus in 18-year-old female with large AV malformation in mesencephalon and third ventricle (arrow). Fatal hemorrhage in mesencephalon

Fig. 5. Large temporal AV malformation extending to lateral ventricle and cisterna ambiens in 39-year-old man

Fig. 6. Multiple AV angiomas in temporal white matter and mesencephalon of 60-year-old male

Fig. 7. Venous angioma in deep cerebellum and pons which had ruptured into fourth ventricle in man aged 48 years

Table II

Fig. 8. Varix-like venous angioma in medulla of 58-year-old male

Figs. 9, 10. Venous angioma with recent hemorrhage in medulla of 20-year-old female. H. & E. $\times$ 40

Fig. 11. Cerebellar hemorrhage in 11-year-old girl with AV angioma

Fig. 12. Varix of great vein of Galen (v) with multiple AV shunts to cerebral vessels and generalized angiodysplasia, hydrocephalus and cystic encephalopathy in newborn male with cardiac failure

Fig. 13. Cryptic AV angioma in choroid plexus of lateral ventricle in 47-year-old male with lethal hemorrhage into parietal lobe. Van Gieson $\times$ 30

Fig. 14. Biopsy specimen of AV malformation in choroid plexus of lateral ventricle in boy aged 11 years with acute cerebral hemorrhage. Van Gieson $\times$ 60

Fig. 15. Venous angioma in choroid plexus of lateral ventricle in 3-year-old boy who died of acute cerebral hemorrhage. H. 5 E. $\times$ 48

Table II

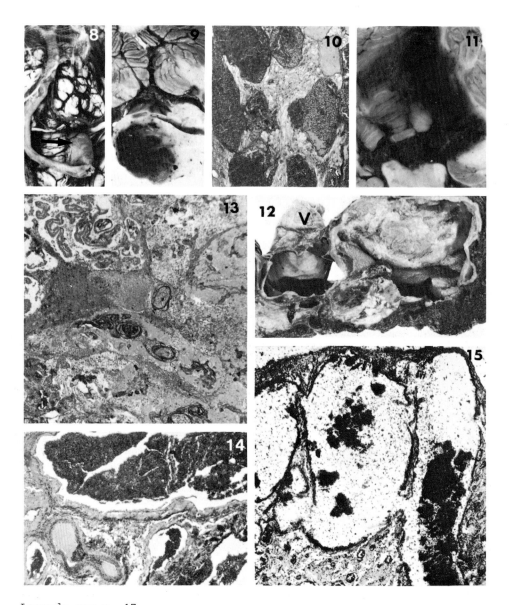

Legends see p. 17

18

Discussion on Chapter I

PIA: It is somewhat disappointing from the viewpoint of a neurosurgeon to see those angiomas which are situated in the brainstem itself, and unfortunately even in these days we must say that we are unable to operate upon them.

FEINDEL: Could we just ask a small point from Dr. Jellinger? A misnomer is often applied to the Galenic malformations. They are called aneurysms of the vein of Galen. They really are just arteriovenous malformations, I take it?

JELLINGER: The so-called varix or aneurysm of the vein of Galen is a large dilatation of this vein, but in the majority of cases, particularly in children, it is almost constantly associated with an arteriovenous malformation. I think there are extremely rare cases where we can say it is a simple varix.

WALTER: (to Dr. Jellinger) I am surprised by the large number of venous angiomas in your report. They were previously considered by pathologists to be an extreme rarity.

JELLINGER: That is a very difficult question, but for the clinician of no great importance. I think it is of decisive importance for the pathologist to get enough material for examinations, because he is often unable to say whether the vessels are to be classified as arteries or veins. Therefore the simplest possible classification should be used.

LAPRAS: We prefer to call the syndrome you have mentioned that of Blanc-Bonnet-De Chaume. I think we were the first to describe angiomas of the brainstem associated with an angioma of the retina and an angioma of the face. As to the nomenclature, we call the malformations of the vein of Galen aneurysms, but I am sure they are arteriovenous malformations.

JELLINGER: I think it is very difficult to decide whether the dilatation or aneurysm as well as the cardiac failure is primary or secondary. This may be particularly the case in some of the elder patients.

JOHNSON: We have had experience of three cases of so-called gyral angiomas. The first patient presented with a cerebello-pontine-angle syndrome and Myodil ventriculography showed a shift of the fourth ventricle. This patient was operated upon, and the lesion found was a large "venous aneurysm". After the operation the vertebral and left carotid angiograms were done and were negative. A right carotid angiogam was positive, showing filling of a large venous lake. The operation on this patient consisted of exploring the tentorium and the petrous bone widely and dividing all the meningeal vessels entering into this lake of blood. The next case was a man with a filling defect in the fourth ventricle on Myodil ventriculography. At operation again a large venous lake of blood arising from the floor of the fourth ventricle was found. The vertebral angiogram was negative, but the venous angioma filled from the right external carotid. In the third case, a similar lesion in the right cerebellar hemisphere was supplied from a meningeal branch of the vertebral artery. There were two veins draining into the torcula, entering it very close together. On the left side venous blood was draining in, on the right side the vein was arterialized. The latter vein was fed through a meningeal vessel running up in the posterior fossa dura, entering the torcula and emptying into this vein, so that the blood flow in it was reserved. This may explain some of these enormous venous dilatations.

NADJMI: As a neuroradiologist I would like to mention a group of angiomas, which morphologically are seldom seen. They are meningeal venous angiomas fed only by meningeal arteries and their venous drainage appears immediately. We previously called them venous angiomas, but after subtraction we were able to see feeding arteries coming from the artery of Bernascone or the petrous part of the carotid. They have to be looked for. I think we should solve this problem by admitting the existence of angiomas fed exclusively by meningeal arteries.

JELLINGER: The pathologist has to be cautious about admitting this type of angioma, but I think that better angiographic techniques will alter the relationship between venous and arteriovenous malformations in favor of the latter.

Chapter II
Clinical Aspects

The Epidemiology and Clinical Course of Arteriovenous Malformations

G. PERRET

D e f i n i t i o n

The Cooperative Study of Intracranial Aneurysms and Subarachnoid Hemorrhage (1) indicated that surgical or nonsurgical treatment depended on the age of the patient, size and location of the lesion, presence or absence of hemorrhage, and the severity of illness at the time of the treatment. Technical operability was determined essentially by the size and site of the lesion. Of the 453 Arteriovenous Malformations (AVM) in this study, 50% were not treated surgically. Of 36 nonbleeding AVM without seizures, 24 were not operated upon; of 101 nonbleeding AVM with seizures, 83 were not operated upon; of 281 bleeding AVM, 103 were not operated upon; of 31 infratentorial AVM, 2 were considered inoperable, and 14 were not operated upon. However, no light is shed on what really is an inoperable lesion, nor why this large number was not surgically treated.

What is an inoperable AVM? Inoperability of AVM essentially depends on its size and location. Cerebral midline malformations, those involving the ventricles, the paraventricular structures, the basal ganglia, the thalamus, the hypothalamus, the choroid plexus, the splenium of the corpus callosum, the midbrain, the cerebral peduncles, the pons, the medulla oblongata, the anterior-superior cerebellum, and the upper cervical cord are usually considered inoperable (2, 3, 4). Other lesions which may not be operable are malformations which involve a large portion of the convexity, especially of the dominant cerebral hemisphere or of the medial surface of one or both hemispheres (3), supplied by branches of 2, 3, or 4 main arteries, and which drain into the deep cerebral venous system as well as into the convexity sinuses. Anatomically one must remember that many AVMs have their arterial components on or just below the cortex, but drain into paraventricular venous channels. Thus, the malformation has a wedge shaped configuration with the base at the cortex and the apex at the edge of the lateral ventricle (5). Such a configuration will render inoperable some anomalies involving the Sylvian fissure of the dominant hemisphere or the Rolandic areas. Three vessel stereoscopic angiography is always necessary for diagnosis in the patient with subarachnoid hemorrhage or when an AVM is suspected by clinical or dynamic brain scan examination, as anomalies of the circle of Willis are frequent. Only few published reports precisely describe the origin of the blood supply to the AVM or its drainage (6).

Of the 453 AVM reported in the Cooperative Study (1), 81 or 18% were intraventricular or paraventricular involving the midline cerebral structures. Of these, 34 were on the right side, 31 on the left; 16 were bilateral. Eleven or 2% were in or around the brain stem and 21 or 5% in the cerebellum. Three lesions were reported to involve one entire hemisphere. No mention is made of the size of the other hemispheric malformations, and no information is available about the arterial blood supply and venous drainage, nor reasons for their operability or inoperability.

337 or 61% of all AVMs reported by the Cooperative Study (1) had a history of subarachnoid hemorrhage. 24% of the bleeding malformations had manifested themselves by the age of 30. The hemorrhage was fatal in 10%. Recurrent hemorrhages occurred in 23% of the cases. The interval between bleeding episodes varied from a few days to over 20 years.

Convulsive seizures were the presenting symptoms in 24% of cases without antecedent hemorrhage. 70% of the patients who had seizures did not have hemorrhage during the 7 years of the study, and 88% of patients with hemorrhage had no seizures.

The literature contains no report dealing exclusively with inoperable AVMs. Most surgeons prefer to write about the operable cases, about their success in treating large and frightening lesions, but little is written about the surgically inaccessible ones. Others discuss series of untreated AVMs, but without evaluating them in regard to their operability (7, 8, 9). These considerations led to the present review of 98 AVMs diagnosed and treated on the neurosurgical service of the University of Iowa during the past 10 years. They included 52 females and 46 males. The ratio was 1.1 females to 1 male, which is a reverse of the usually reported ratio.

Table 1. AVM Iowa 1963-1973

Age	Male	Female	Total	Hemorrhage Male	Female	Total
0-9	3	1	4	2	–	2
10-19	6	10	16	5	8	13
20-29	7	19	26	5	11	16
30-39	14	6	20	6	1	7
40-49	4	6	10	3	2	5
50-59	5	3	8	1	1	2
60-69	6	4	10	3	2	5
70+	1	3	4	1	–	1
Total	46	52	98	26	25	51

Table 1 shows the relation between sex, age, and hemorrhage. 54% of these AVMs were symptomatic before the age of 30, 65% between the ages of 10 and 39. Hemorrhages occurred in 51% of them, in an equal number of males and females. 62% of the bleeding AVMs had manifested themselves by the age of 30. The hemorrhage was fatal in 2%. Recurrent hemorrhage occurred in 11% of the cases or 22% of the bleeding malformations. The interval between bleeding episodes varied from 10 days to 26 years, with an average of 11 years. Twelve intracranial aneurysms were angiographically demonstrated in 7 of the patients who bled.

Convulsions occurred in 37% of the patients. 14% of the 98 patients
had both seizures and hemorrhages. 62% of patients with convulsions
never bled, and 27% of patients with bleeding malformations had seizures. Convulsions were more frequent in males, and were present before the age of 20 in 27% of the patients. Headache was the most frequent symptom (52%). It nearly always accompanied hemorrhage. 46 patients had neurologic deficits when first examined; the most common
being visual fields defects, hemiparesis, speech difficulties, and
sensory disturbances. Cranial bruit was heard in 22 patients (11 with
cranial and extracranial AVM and 11 with intracranial lesions). Mental
disturbances were uncommon (4%). Eleven bleeding patients were unresponsive when admitted to the hospital; all had intraparenchymal hematomas.

In our series, 37% of the patients were operated upon. 22 of these 37
patients had large parenchymal hematomas, which necessitated surgical
intervention. 12 of them remained responsive after the hemorrhage. In
the younger age group, the hematoma frequently resulted from rupture of
small (cryptic) AVMs fed by only one artery. 36% of the patients who
presented minor symptoms or had convulsions only were treated conservatively and in an additional 27% the lesion was considered inoperable.

The mortality rate in this angiographically diagnosed series of patients
with AVMs was 8%; 2 from cerebral hemorrhage, 2 following surgical intervention, 1 from cerebral infarction, 2 from lung carcinoma, 1 of a
gunshot wound. Thus, in only 4 was death related to the AVM. This represents a mortality of 4% of the bleeding malformations, and a 5.5%
operative mortality. However, during the same period, 4% of the University of Iowa autopsy population or 135 patients had AVM; 81 males
and 54 females with ages from 1 day to 83 years. Only 20 patients
showed evidence of hemorrhage from the AVM; 15 of them died of a massive hemorrhage, most of them from small cryptic intraparenchymal malformations. Their age ranged from 1 day to 65 years. In 13 of these
patients dying from massive intracerebral hemorrhages, the diagnosis
was not made before death as they were moribund when admitted to the
hospital. In the other 2, the diagnosis was made by angiography (see
above). Thus, the overall mortality rate from hemorrhage from AVMs is
11%, which coincides with other statistics.

C l i n i c a l   C o u r s e

Of the 27 patients with inoperable lesions, 12 were females, and 15
males, aged from 7 to 67 years (12 below the age of 30). Ten (37%)
AVMs were intraventricular or paraventricular involving the basal ganglia in 5 patients, the thalamus bilaterally in 3, and the ventricle
and the choroid plexus in two. Four were in or on the brain stem involving the midbrain in one, the fourth ventricle in one and the upper
cervical cord in one. Two were in the midline over the superior surface of the cerebellum. Six convexity AVMs were considered inoperable
because of their size; another 5 were situated over the medial aspect
of the parietal lobes, involving both hemispheres and the corpus callosum in 3. The blood supply to these malformations came from 2 main
arteries in 15 cases, 3 arteries in 5, 4 arteries in 6, and in one
case the arterial supply could not be fully identified, because the
malformation covered the medulla oblongata and the cervical cord. One
or both posterior cerebral arteries were frequently involved together
with the anterior choroidal and peri-callosal arteries. Supply from
all 3, - anterior, middle, and posterior - cerebral arteries was fre-

quent in the larger convexity lesions. They drained into the deep venous system and occasionally into dural sinuses. Three of the cases were associated with intracranial aneurysms (1 case had 3 aneurysms), and one with an aneurysmal dilatation of the vein of Galen. 50% of these malformations bled. Nine patients presented with an initial hemorrhage while 5 had recurrent hemorrhages after intervals from the previous hemorrhage of 5, 8, 18, 24, and 26 years (Table 2). It seems that the rate of recurrent hemorrhage is greater in this group than in the rest of the AVMs, (36% vs 22%), although the overall rate of hemorrhage remains the same.

Table 2. Inoperable AVM

Age	Number	Hemorrhage	Convulsions	Hemorrhage & Convulsions	Neurologic Deficits
0-9	1	–	1	–	1
10-19	5	4	–	–	4
20-29	6	3	3	1	2
30-39	8	3	4	1	4
40-49	4	2	2	1	2
50-59	2	1	2	1	1
60+	1	1	–	–	1
Total	27	14	12	4	15

Only one of these patients had a small angiographically demonstrable hematoma. Except for posterior fossa AVM, the hemorrhage was more likely to occur in the ventricular system, but was not fatal. Convulsive seizures occurred in 12 (44%) patients; they were focal in 7. Four of the patients had hemorrhage and seizures. The convulsions preceded the time of diagnosis by one to 23 years.

Headache was the main complaint in 17 patients, including 11 who bled. Neurologic deficits were present in 15 patients and included paresis, sensory loss, visual loss, cranial nerve signs, and hydrocephalus in 2 cases. They were more frequent and perhaps more severe than in the usual convexity AVM. Five of the 27 patients had neither convulsions nor hemorrhage. Three of them presented initially with neurological deficit and 2 with headache only. Intracranial bruit was heard in 5, and one patient became unresponsive immediately after the hemorrhage.

Over a 10 year period, 1963-1973, frequent checkup examinations showed that of 21 patients who were working or going to school, 7 were asymptomatic, 11 had mild neurologic deficits, and in 9 the convulsions were adequately controlled. Four patients were unable to work because of severe neurologic deficit, uncontrolable seizures or mental deficits. In this group no patient died of hemorrhage; 1 patient died of lung carcinoma 30 years after the onset of focal seizures and progressive left hemiparesis; 1 patient was lost for followup.

Comments

The behavior of AVM is unpredictable. The size of the lesion is not related to the presenting symptoms. The prognosis following hemorrhage does not correlate with the location of the lesion nor the age of the patient. Af BJÖRKESTEN and TROUPP (6) and others (2, 3, 7, 10) are unable to find any factors that point to a particularly good or bad prognosis. Most authors agree that the best treatment for bleeding AVM is radical excision of the lesion (13). Excluding some midline supra- and infratentorial malformations, most large lesions are surgically accessible (12). They are not inoperable; however, the risk of the surgical procedure is often unwarranted in the presence of minor symptoms and after consideration of all of the possible neurologic deficits which may follow operation and incapacitate the patient (3, 13). This is especially true in the presence of intra- or paraventricular lesions or brain stem lesions.

Operability also depends upon the youth, the experience, or the inexperience of the surgeon.

S u m m a r y

1. Inoperable AVMs are defined as lesions involving the intra- or paraventricular areas, the brain stem and large hemispheric convexity anomalies. 2. Inoperable AVM represent approximately 27% of all AVMs. They occur at any age, predominantely in the younger age group. They bleed more frequently than convexity lesions, but are usually not fatal. 3. These lesions are usually fed by 2, 3, or 4 main arteries and drain into the deep venous system. 4. In our series, 80% of the patients with such lesions were either asymptomatic or had mild neurologic deficit, and were able to work.

R e f e r e n c e s

1. PERRET, G. E., NISHIOKA, H.: Arteriovenous Malformations. In: Sahs, A. L., Perret, G. E., Locksley, H. B., Nishioka, H. (eds.): Intracranial Aneurysms and Subarachnoid Hemorrhage; A Cooperative Study. Philadelphia & Toronto: J. B. Lippincott 1969.

2. GILLINGHAM, J.: Arteriovenous Malformations of the Head. Edinb. Med. Journ. 60, 305-319 (1953).

3. MCKISSOCK, W., HANKINSON, J.: The Surgical Treatment of Supratentorial Angiomas. First International Congress of Neurosurgery, Brussels, p. 223-228 (1957).

4. FRENCH, L. A., CHOU, S. N.: Conventional Methods of Treating Intracranial Arteriovenous Malformations. Prog. Neurol. Surg. 3, p. 274-319. Basel: Karger & Chicago: Year Book 1969.

5. KAPLAN, H. A., ARONSON, S. M., BROWDER, E. J.: Vascular Malformations of the Brain; An Anatomical Study. J. Neurosurg. 18, 630-635 (1961).

6. AF BJÖRKESTEN, G., TROUPP, H.: Arteriovenous Malformations of the Brain. Acta Psych. & Neurol. Scand. 34, 429-437 (1959).

7. MACKENZIE, I.: The Clinical Presentation of the Cerebral Angioma. Brain. 76, 184-214 (1953).

8. POTTER, J. M.: Angiomatous Malformations of the Brain; Their Nature & Prognosis. Ann. Roy. Coll. Surg. Engl. 16, 227-242 (1955).

9. SVIEN, H. J., MCCRAE, J. A.: Arteriovenous Malformations of the Brain. J. Neurosurg. 23, 23-28 (1965).

10. KELLY, D. L., ALEXANDER, E., DAVIS, C. H., MAYNARD, D. C.: Intracranial Arteriovenous Malformations; Clinical Review & Evaluation of Brain Scans. J. Neurosurg. 31, 422-428 (1969).

11. SEDZIMIR, C. B., ROBINSON, J.: Intracranial Hemorrhage in Children & Adolescents. J. Neurosurg. 38, 269-281 (1973).

12. MILLETTI, M.: Discussion on Supratentorial Angiomas. First International Congress of Neurosurgery, Brussels, p.249-251 (1957).

13. FRENCH, L. A., STORY, J. L.: Cerebrovascular Malformations. Clin. Neurosurg. 11, 9. 171-182 (1964).

The Influence of the Type and Localization of the Angioma on the Clinical Syndrome

W. WALTER

The attempt to show any relationship between the clinical picture, the size and type of angioma as well as its location, and the indication for operation is limited right from the outset by the fact that the newer operative procedures have not been considered in the evaluation of what were previously inoperable angiomas. In other words, the operability of angiomas by means of stereotaxy, cryosurgery and embolisation is not discussed here because the patients in our series have not been treated by these methods. We will begin from the baseline of previously used indication for a direct surgical approach where the optimal therapeutic goal is the complete removal of the angioma. In addition the ligation of supplying vessels following the exposure of the angioma will also be considered.

In a survey of the entire case material of TÖNNIS and SCHIEFER, a series of 281 arteriovenous angiomas was reviewed. For the sake of clarity, I will begin by giving a brief description of the anatomical pathology and histopathology. Generally, the clinician deals only with the arteriovenous angioma. Cavernous angiomas are much less common, being often an incidental finding, and coming to our attention only when a hemorrhage occurs. The same is true for telangiectasias which are similar to arteriovenous angiomas as far as the histopathology is concerned, but through which there is not the typical arteriovenous shunt.

The so-called venous angioma will always present some difficulties in that there is a gradual transition from the wide venous angiomatous spaces to the so-called varices of the brain. Such venous angiomas whose histological picture is characterized by the chiefly venous structure of the blood-containing spaces may be found partly in the Rolandic fissure and partly in the dura mater. The so-called aneurysm of the vein of Galen, consisting of large venous malformations of the vein of Galen, should possibly be grouped with this type of angioma.

Let me begin with a few words about terminology: The term midline angioma carried the implication of being inoperable before the recent introduction of the above-mentioned methods. Midline angiomas comprise angiomatous malformations located in the medulla oblongata, the pons, the midbrain, the hypothalamus or the mesencephalon. If they are situated in the basal ganglia, they must be present on both sides or at least receive feeding vessels from both sides in order to be a genuine midline tumor (Fig.1).

The angiomas in the posterior fossa are also included here, although there are certainly occasional angiomas located only in the hemisphere or in the cerebellar tonsils so that the term midline angioma is not completely correct. However, angiomas limited to only one cerebellar hemisphere or to only one cerebellar tonsil are rare. As a rule, they cross the midline and must therefore be classified in the above-mentioned group. All angiomas of the posterior fossa that involve the medulla, the pons and the midbrain belong here.

In Table 1 the locations of interest are listed together once more. For these angiomas the indication for operation was limited till now, or there was actually a contraindication to total removal.

Table 1. Location and indication for total removal

Restricted Indication or Contraindication for Total Extirpation

Midline angiomas	medulla, midbrain, diencephalon
Midline angiomas	bilateral in the area of oral brainstem (thalamus, capsula int., pallidum, putamen, claustrum)
Midline angiomas	corpus callosum or interhemispheric fissure, both hemispheres
Unilateral angiomas	lateral ventricle and wall, thalamus, capsula int., pallidum, putamen, claustrum
Unilateral angiomas	huge, in functional important areas

On surveying the literature and studying our own cases, we gained the impression that angiomas in the basal ganglia and the corpus callosum possess certain peculiarities in the clinical presentation. LITVAK, YAHR and RANSOHOFF (2) divided vascular malformations of the midline into 3 groups.

a) Aneurysms of the vein of Galen, which consist of an enlargement of the vein of Galen together with an enlarged straight and confluent sinus with feeding vessels from abnormal branches of the carotid artery or the circle of Willis.

b) Racemose conglomerates of cerebral vessels with dilatation of the deeper draining veins. These vessel conglomerates consist of arteriovenous shunts in the sense of an angioma or a hemangioma lying in the midline or in the deeper cerebral structures and emptying towards the center into veins or into a sinus.

c) Transitional types of arteriovenous shunts of the midline:
   1. Individual vessels, with the exception of the vein of Galen, which empty into a dilated sinus or into veins.
   2. Combinations of midline angiomas with one or more aneurysmally dilated vessels.
   3. Direct arterial shunts into abnormal or dilated venous sinuses.

The demonstration of the individual types is never as clearly deline-
ated as this classification indicates. We have presented it in detail
because the clinical symptomatology of the individual groups may have
certain peculiarities.

In the case of vascular malformations of the midline and those near
the drainage vessels into the great vein of Galen, hydrocephalus may
occur more frequently than with angiomas located in other sites, primarily because of an obstruction to the CSF passage. The literature
indicates that this occlusion is generally caused by compression of
the aqueduct and less by obstruction of the foramen of Monroe.

Angiomas of the basal ganglia, of the corpus callosum and the interhemispheric fissure justify a separate description because their symptomatology differs from that of angiomas in the cerebral hemispheres.
Many authors in the literature have pointed out that epileptic seizures
are relatively rare while hemorrhage is accompanied by hemiparesis in
a high percentage of cases. This is true for our own case material
also. Particularly high is the percentage of cases with a so-called
paralytic presentation, no less than one-third of our own patients
having a slowly developing paresis as the first symptom (Table 2).
Hydrocephalus as a sequel to a hemorrhage or as a sequel to compression
of the aqueduct or of the foramen of Monroe has been mentioned already.
Hemorrhage almost always results in a difficult clinical course since
it almost always leads to an intracerebral hematoma, not infrequently
accompanied by rupture into the ventricle similar to the mechanism
seen in cases of hypertensive hemorrhage. The prognosis is unfavorable.

Table 2. Symptomatology of midline angiomas

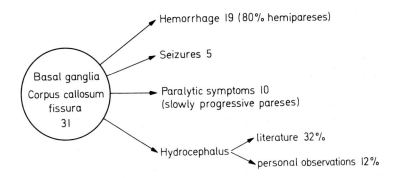

Angiomas of the posterior fossa do not have a symptomatology comparable with angiomas of the cerebral hemispheres. As Table 3 shows, 58
patients with angiomas of the posterior fossa (18 patients from our
own case material and 40 from the literature) were investigated. Of
special note is the fact that subarachnoid hemorrhage does not play
the dominant role it does in the case of angiomas of the cerebral hemispheres. The clinical signs are often those of a space-occupying lesion
in the posterior fossa. Thus it is not surprising that 50% of our own
patients and 30% of the patients in the literature had chronic papil-
loedema without any acute episode indicative of a hemorrhage. The most
common symptoms are headache, vomiting, double vision, dizziness, ataxia and disturbances of coordination. Cranial nerve palsies are also
often found. For example trigeminal neuralgia was found in 11% of all
cases. Epileptic seizures are extremely uncommon in this site. In order

Table 3. Symptomatology of angiomas of the posterior fossa

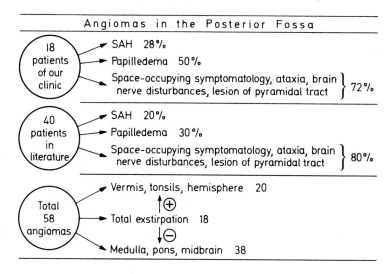

of incidence, symptoms of increased intracranial pressure and of cerebellar involvement are most common. Involvement of the cranial nerves
as well as of the pyramidal tracts occurs whenever either the medulla
and/or the pons or the midbrain were affected. Our own case material
and a review of the literature indicate that total removal is possible
only in those cases where the angioma is limited to the vermis, the
tonsils or the cerebellar hemisphere. The only palliative operation
today consists of a ventriculo-atrial shunt. Follow-up studies on our
patients show that they can survive for years without serious problems.
The last group of our own results to be discussed deals with the so-
called aneurysms of the great vein of Galen, which is the subject of
much discussion particularly in the Anglo-Saxon literature (Table 4),
(the last review was compiled by AMACHER and SHILLITO (1). The first
extensive survey was made by LITVAK and his team. AMACHER and SHILLITO
reported 37 cases in the literature as well as 5 cases of their own.
Our case material contains 3 such cases which should be classified
with this group.

As Table 4 indicates, these aneurysms have been classified according
to their clinical features into the following groups to which we shall
adhere. Group 1 includes children from birth up to the age of 3. The
characteristic symptoms here are a vascular murmur, widening of the
sutures and enlargement of the head, as well as possibly calcification
in the pineal region. Group 2 includes only a few patients. They were
all 1 - 6 months old and were detected because of their cardiac symptomatology, and later because of a slight enlargement of the head. The
third group lay between the 1st and 12th month and were found to have
hydrocephalus in 70% of the cases. Several of these small patients also had seizures. Not a single child had presented with a subarachnoid
hemorrhage. In recent years, the tendency to operate in these cases
has increased.

In the series of 37 patients reported by AMACHER and SHILLITO, 16 were
operated upon, and, of these, 10 survived. Generally the attempt was
made to remove the large venous sack completely. Our own group includes
3 such patients. In one case we were able to remove the large venous

Table 4. Symptomatology of the so-called "aneurysms of the great vein of Galen" - literature 42 patients, personal observations 3 patients (slightly modified from AMACHER and SHILLITO, 1973)

	No. of patients	Symptoms
Group I post-natal	11	cardiac symptoms intracranial bruit
Group II post-natal or 1-6 months	4	little cardiac symptoms, and marked increase of head circumference
Group III 1-12 months	23	increase of head circumference, vessel bruit, hydrocephalus
Group IV 2-27 years	7	headaches, calcifications in the pineal region, hydrocephalus, paralytic pareses

sack entirely. The child had come to our attention because of the signs of slowly increasing intracranial pressure leading to optic nerve atrophy. In the second case, atrio-ventricular drainage with a Spitz-Holder valve was instituted. The patient has now survived for several years. Although we were able to demonstrate the vascular malformation in the scintigram in the third case, death occurred before angiography could be performed. As the pathology specimen shows, typical hydrocephalus had developed already. The child was 14 months old.

We studied the more than 250 angiograms of arteriovenous angiomas at our disposal with respect to their symptomatology and the operative success as far as total removal was concerned, and we had the impression that the type of angioma may also play a special role. This is especially true for angiomas of the cerebral hemispheres which necessitate a particularly careful analysis of the indications for operation because they are frequently situated in areas of important cerebral function. As Table 5 indicates, we have attempted to classify angiomas into four distinct types although we are aware of the fact that there is a gradual transition from one group to the other and that clear delineation is seldom possible. The indication for the total removal of an angioma in an area of important cerebral function is present when the angioma is compact and clearly circumscribed, and drained by a single hypertrophied vein or only a few drainage veins limited to the vicinity of the angioma. Here serial angiography is of decisive importance for it permits the actual delineation of the angioma in the various phases. In the second group, we include the more diffuse angiomas, the differences being particularly masked in the capillary phase, which at the same time have only one or a few enlarged drainage veins. Today these angiomas can also be removed relatively well using microsurgical techniques without additional severe damage to brain tissue. The third group contains diffuse angiomas with numerous, enlarged draining veins, some of which are well developed far away from the angioma and not infrequently have the appearance of typical venous dilatations. Especially in the late capillary or late venous phases, one gains the impression of a cerebral "varicosis", if you will allow the use of this term here. In the fourth group we include the previously discussed, so-called aneurysms of the great vein of Galen. As we said at the beginning, these angiomas may probably best be grouped more or less with the venous angiomas. Recently surgical procedures attempting the total removal of these angiomas have become more frequent. In our opinion the methods of embolisation or stereotaxy are unlikely to be useful.

Table 5. Type of angioma and operability

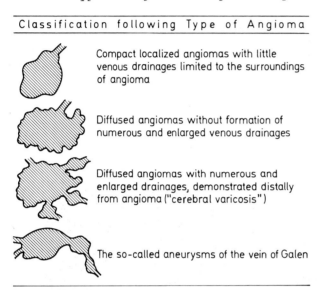

Classification following Type of Angioma	
	Compact localized angiomas with little venous drainages limited to the surroundings of angioma
	Diffused angiomas without formation of numerous and enlarged venous drainages
	Diffused angiomas with numerous and enlarged drainages, demonstrated distally from angioma ("cerebral varicosis")
	The so-called aneurysms of the vein of Galen

These remarks are by no means intended to dictate what can be operated on and what not. We are aware of the fact that it is almost impossible to make firm predictions about what may be possibly severe post-operative neurological deficit. Again and again, one finds that angiomas in the central region, for example, which had led one to fear a hemiparalysis, can be removed without severe disturbance and that on the other hand, angiomas near the central region may lead to very severe neurological deficits after operative intervention. This discussion is only intended to initiate an exchange of experiences about the total removal of angiomas. Furthermore, those angiomas which are not accessible to total removal have been presented. The methods of cryosurgery and embolisation will considerably facilitate our thoughts about indication for operation.

R e f e r e n c e s

1. AMACHER, A. L., SHILLITO, J.: The syndromes and surgical treatment of aneurysms of the great vein of Galen. J. Neurosurgery, 39, 89-98 (1973).

2. LITVAK, J., YAHR, M. D., RANSOHOFF, J.: Aneurysms of the great vein of Galen and midline cerebral arteriovenous anomalies. J. Neurosurgery, 17, 945-954, 1960.

3. TÖNNIS, W., WALTER, W., BROCK, M.: Die Totalextirpation intracerebraler arteriovenöser Angiome bei Lokalisation in funktionell wichtigen Hirnarealen. Beitr. Neurochir. H. 11. Leipzig: Barth 1966.

4. TÖNNIS, W., WALTER, W.: Differentialdiagnose, Klinik und Behandlung
   der cerebralen Gefäßmißbildungen. Zu: Biologie und Klinik des Zentralnervensystems. Basel: Sandoz 1967.

5. WALTER, W.: Klinik, Diagnostik und operative Behandlung der intracraniellen Gefäßmißbildungen und nicht-traumatischen Blutungen.
   Habilitationsschrift Köln 1965.

6. WALTER, W., BISCHOF, W.: Klinik und operative Behandlung der arte-
   riösen Angiome des Stammhirns bzw. der sog. Mittellinienangiome.
   Neurochirurgia, 9, 150-166 (1966).

7. WALTER, W., SCHEFFLER, G., BISCHOF, W.: Klinik und Therapie der arteriovenösen Angiome im Bereich der hinteren Schädelgrube. Dtsch.
   Zeitschr. S. Nervenheilk. 191, 39-73 (1967).

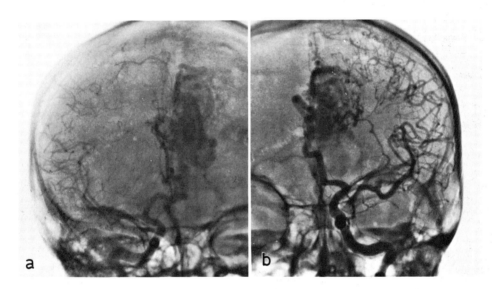

Fig. 1 a and b. Typical midline angioma filled from both sides

Discussion on Chapter II

Presentation: PERRET (Epidemiology and Clinical Course)

Presentation: WALTER (Influence of the Type and Location of an Angioma
on the Clinical Syndrome)

KOHLMEYER: I wonder whether the combination of angiomas and aneurysms is really so rare. Among more than hundred intracerebral hemorrhages we found this combination on three occasions.

WALTER: In reviewing the literature we found 42 such cases.

PIA: We had 5 or 6 cases among 120 intracranial angiomas, and all of them had bled. It was very difficult to decide whether the hemorrhage arose from the angioma or from the aneurysm. In most of the cases the angioma was the source of the hemorrhage.

PERRET: In the cooperative study of about 500 arteriovenous malformations we found 56 cases with aneurysms, this gives an incidence of about 10%.

SCHÜRMANN: We had 3 aneurysms in a series of 80 angiomas. In one case we missed the aneurysm, and after the angioma had been excised we had to clip the aneurysm, which was the source of the hemorrhage at a second operation. As to midbrain angiomas we successfully clipped in one of our patients the feeding vessels from the anterior chorioideal, both pericallosals, the Sylvian, and the posterior chorioideal arteries in three operative sessions, and we diminished the size of the malformation considerably. Control angiography showed late and prolonged filling. We were pleased with ourselves, but two years later the patient had to be readmitted in a decerebrate state due to severe recurrent ventricular hemorrhage.

RIECHERT: We have had two cases of the combination of an angioma with a tumor. The first one bled 11 times and we were repeatedly unable to demonstrate the angioma angiographically. At autopsy, a cherry-sized spongioblastoma with an angioma was found. Our second patient had a massive hemorrhage followed by long-standing loss of consciousness and hemiplegia. Stereotactically I was unable to extirpate the angioma in the caudoventral part of the thalamus. Biopsy of the surrounding softened cerebral tissue revealed an oligodendroglioma. Of course, we must not confuse these rare combiantions of tumor and angioma with a vascularized tumor.

AGNOLI: In some cases of extracranial angiomas a spontaneous cure has been observed. Has anybody had a similar experience with intracranial angiomas and a spontaneous cure demonstrated on angiography?

WALTER (to AGNOLI): We have seen three cases of so-called micro-angiomas which caused hemorrhage and which we managed conservatively. Repeat angiography after three weeks did not demonstrate the angioma. However, I have never seen this happen in cases of large angiomas.

TZONOS: I would like to add a comment on the case of Dr. Riechert's. In children with a spongioblastoma of the midline angiomatous malformations have been demonstrated histologically several times. I think there is a type of spongioblastoma with an angiomatous component, which I have seen on three or four occasions. Even on a retrospective evaluation of the angiograms the differential diagnosis between a tumor and angioma or a vascularized tumor was impossible.

LOEW: (to the question of AGNOLI) We had a child with a severe subarachnoid, and probably intracerebral hemorrhage from an angioma of the left thalamus. We did not operate, and the child survived with a slowly improving hemiparesis. Two years later, no more than a middle-sized angioma could be demonstrated. Thus spontaneous thrombosis at the time of hemorrhage must be assumed.

To the question of RIECHERT: We have seen at our clinic a case of an oligodendroglioma of the right hemisphere and an angioma of the left. The patient was operated upon for the tumor and died four or five years later from a recurrence. The angioma never caused any symptomatology. I think that in this case there were two clinical syndromes independent of each other. Statistically two different pathologies may rarely occur spontaneously in one patient.

DJINDJIAN: I think that it is important to discriminate between an angioma and an angiectasis. In my opinion the information is lacking; if you have a tumor in one cerebral hemisphere , you should - in order to obtain full information - perform 2 external carotid, 2 internal carotid, 2 vertebral, cervical, and descending cervical angiograms. Actually by the femoral route you could always carry out these examinations in one session.

PERRET: There are several cases of glioma associated with venous malformation reported in the literature. Recently we had a case of a 37-year-old urologist who had convulsions for three years. Angiographically there was an arteriovenous malformation of the right paramedian posterior frontal region. He was advised by several neurosurgeons not to be operated upon. 3 years later he developed visual disturbances and had bilateral chronic high-grade papilledema. We repeated the angiograms which showed a big arteriovenous malformation. We thought, because of the clinical symptoms that we were dealing with an angioblastic type of a meningioma. At operation we found an arteriovenous malformation surrounded by an infiltrating glioma, grade III. We do not know whether the tumor was present in an early stage three years previously or not.

SCHEPELMANN: I would like to mention another way in which it is possible to miss the association of an arteriovenous angioma and an aneurysm. We had a case of a huge cerebral angioma in which four vessel angiography was performed in order to consider the operability of the lesion. The patient was operated upon, and the postoperative angiogram showed a cherry-sized aneurysm of the vertebral artery, which did not fill before. I think that the preoperative non-filling was caused

by the arteriovenous shunt. There are probably more cases of arteriovenous malformation associated with aneurysms than are recognized, but
because of the shunt the aneurysm is not demonstrated.

PIA: We have heard a lot about the size, type, and location of angiomas.
Now let us discuss the clinical picture and the decisive role it should
play in the indication for surgery. For instance there may be a case
of an operable angioma, which has never bled and causes only mild symptoms, e.g. seizures from time to time. Let us talk about those cases
in which operation appears possible, but the indication for surgery is
not clear. On the other hand there are cases where symptoms clearly
contraindicate surgery. I remind you of Olivecrona's statement that
long-standing epilepsy is not of great concern to the patient.

PERRET: It is my opinion and that of our group that an operable lesion
should not always be operated upon. We think that, if an operable lesion presents no symptoms or few symptoms, no neurological deficits,
and only convulsions, the patient does not benefit much from an operation. It has been shown that many of the arteriovenous malformations,
who, when diagnosed, have never bled, will not bleed. Neurologic deficit may not increase and the convulsions, although they may become
more frequent, are still controllable with anticonvulsive medication.
I think it is important to consider when you operate on a lesion, which
is operable, whether you are not going to create neurological deficits,
which the patient did not have, and whether or not you are going to
increase the severity and the frequency of convulsions. This has been
reported by a good number of authors.

KUHLENDAHL: I would like to point out the importance of the age factor.
We all know patients with angiomas who were asymptomatic for many years,
then started to have symptoms at the age of 50 - 60 years and developed
a progressive hemiparesis. I doubt if one can say that young asymptomatic patients should not be operated upon. The factor of the personal
operative experience of the surgeon plays also an important role. I
do not think that we can standardize these indications.

LAPRAS: I agree with Dr. PERRET, but I think that when an angioma presents signs and symptoms while the patient is still young, we can as-
sume that its evolution will be more rapid than if the angioma mani-
fests itself later. So we think that there is a very strong indication
for surgery in young patients.

JOHNSON: Benign angiomas are not always so benign as they seem to be.
We have had two patients who had fatal hemorrhages in late life. One
I remember very well was a solicitor, and his only symptom was that
frequently when he was writing, his pen would just go off the page.
That was the limit of his epilepsy. He had a fatal hemorrhage at the
age of 60 and he had a very operable angioma. Just two other points
on sympatomatology. As Dr. Kuhlendahl says, these patients can deteriorate, and they can deteriorate mentally. I think that this is very
important. Some of them take psychiatric opinions, and the psychiatrist
does not always associate their mental changes with this change in
blood flow in the brain. Another symptom we found, that demanded operation, was trigeminal neuralgia. The angiomas of the upper surface
of the cerebellum can cause intolerable pain.

LUESSENHOP (in reply to the question of DJINDJIAN, whether one should
embolize asymptomatic angiomas): Only on one occasion very early in our
experience have we embolized a patient who was asymptomatic. But I
would like only to add this point: a young person knows he has an arteriovenous malformation. He is intelligent enough to know that he can

bleed, although he may remain almost asymptomatic, and he wants to be cured. I certainly think there are many indications for operation on this lesion, if it is very easily operated upon and very small. Likewise the risk is very small.

RIECHERT: We have discussed two questions so far: whether one should operate upon patients who have epilepsy as the only symptom, and whether progressive mental changes are an indication for operation. Together with ZÜLCH we once analysed patients with epilepsy, and we demonstrated that such patients can develop severe mutual deterioration, become asocial, and unable to work. Before we answer the question we have to prove whether the operation can stop mental deterioration in patients with epilepsy and whether they can be improved. We must take into consideration that every epileptic seizure constitutes a danger for the function of the brain as a whole.

WALTER: 60% of patients who had epilepsy before the total extirpation of an angioma was performed continued to have seizures after surgery. However, in the majority of cases there were less in number and severity. I think that the total extirpation of an angioma does not have any considerable influence on the incidence of seizures.

PIA: I think this is a very important point that must influence the indication for surgery and one which we should keep in mind.

LOEW: We have learned this morning that about 30% of angiomas with minor symptoms cause hemorrhage, and about 10% of all angiomas do bleed. What is important is the mortality of these hemorrhages. It means that 3% of all patients harboring angiomas with minor symptoms, which may be diagnosed by chance, run the risk of dying without operation. We compared this risk with the risk of operation. An easily operable angioma will have an operative risk of less than 3%, but if it is a difficult angioma, I think it better not to operate upon it.

SCHÜRMANN: In my opinion a patient with an angioma is a prospective bleeder, and we must operate, since he can bleed in one or two years. Then we have to ask ourselves why we have not done the operation at a time when it was not so difficult to do.

Chapter III
Angiographical Aspects

The Influence of Modern Angiographic Techniques

H. VOGELSANG

The question whether neuro-surgical intervention is indicated or feasible in the case of a cerebral arteriovenous angioma is nowadays determined to a large extent - depending on the location of the angioma -
by the angiographic findings. During the past 20 years serial angiography and subtraction techniques have brought about important progress in the field of neurological diagnosis. A further advance is the
possibility of a better demonstration of the vertebro-basilar system
by means of the retrograde method via the brachial artery or with the
aid of selective techniques using a femoral catheter. Over a period
of many years success has been achieved in the adequate demonstration
of angiomas in the infratentorial and supratentorial areas. Parallel
with this, there has been a widening of the basis of indication for
operation. The further development of neuro-surgical techniques - here
mention might be made of the operation microscope - has extended still
further the indications for operability. It was then asked whether it
might not be possible to obtain a still better demonstration of the
angiomas, their vascular supply and drainage systems. The demand for
adequate angiographic diagnosis is frequently met today by rapid serial angiography. A good and adequate demonstration of all the arteries participating in the cerebral circulatory system must be regarded
as the basic requirement. Thus, a widespread use of the vertebral angiogram has revealed even in case of vascular malformations in the
supratentorial area that the branches of the posterior cerebral artery
are involved to a greater or less high degree in the blood supply of
these angiomas, which are supplied in the main from the carotid system, and may in individual cases constitute the sole source of supply.
As a result of this, special problems in treatment may arise (19). Angiomas with only one or two arteries of supply might well be regarded
as posing no problems with regard to the indications for operation.
The problem becomes more difficult where the angiomas are supplied from
several arteries, possibly from different vascular territories and such
angiomas may be outside the scope of surgery if an unfavorable location
is an additional factor. The way in which the arteries, veins and the
vascular malformations overlie each other in the projections taken
renders exact differentiation difficult. Until now, arterial tributaries with a calibre of less than 300 microns could not be demonstrated
by traditional angiographic methods.

Angiocinematography using 16 or 25 mm films, or large films where necessary, has furnished new information on the arteries supplying angiomas and the circulation in such vascular malformations, this being
due to the rapid picture sequence of 25 - 50 frames per second (2, 3,
5, 11). The routine application of this technique has failed to gain

38

general acceptance, however, because of the size and quality of the pictures and the technical work involved.

The use of 70 or 100 mm films, possibly with the Sircam camera - in conjunction with high-capacity picture amplifiers - has led in the past 2 - 3 years to distinct progress being made in the field of angiocinematographic diagnosis. The quality of the pictures is now comparable with that of serial angiograms. The process of development is the same as with any other X-ray film. It is also possible to carry out subtraction. The picture speed (up to 4 to 6 per second) is adequate. In the diagnosis of angiomas this method is an improvement.

In assessing the indication for surgical intervention in cerebral angiomas the value of detail angiography i.e. the direct X-ray magnification of serial angiograms is to be rated more highly. Thanks to modern X-ray technology it is now possible to use small focusses of 0.3 x 0.3 or 0.1 x 0.1 mm with high loading in a serial manner. As a result of this, direct X-ray magnification has become possible in serial angiography without loss of clearness. Thanks to the geometrical enlargement it is now possible to recognize objects on the film which were not visible on normal films owing to lack of sharpness of detail. In other words, we find an improvement in the definition of an object which, on a conventional film, is either not demonstrated at all, or if so, only poorly (4, 9, 10). With a 0.3 mm focus the magnification factor of 2.25 proved optimal. Vessels with a lumen of 150 microns in diameter are clearly recognizable. Examination with 0.1 focus tubes showed that with a magnification factor of 4 a good representation of the vessels with a lumen of 80 microns can be achieved (17). Magnification techniques in conjunction with rapid serial angiography and subtraction are able to furnish us today with substantially better information on arteriovenous angiomas.

Further differentiation of the vascular components of the angioma is made possible by the method of cerebral angiotomography, i.e. the combined use of angiography and simultaneous multilayer tomography. Reports on experiences in aneurysms and in the diagnosis of tumors are available (inter alia from ALLCOCK (1); GADO and BULL (7); GERHARDT and OLDENKOTT (8); NADJMI and PÖSCHMANN (12); OLDENKOTT and GERHARDT (13); PIEPGRAS et al. (14); PIEPGRAS and KAMMERER (15); ROSA (16); WAPPENSCHMIDT (18)) and have confirmed the value of this method. For the purposes of angiotomographic examination any all-purpose cranial X-ray machine on which a simultaneous tomography cassette can be mounted is suitable. Also currently offered on the market is a tomography cassette changer (Angiostratix made by Messrs. CGR). The pictures made by this method are of good quality as regards the vessels and their course. A further advantage of angiotomography lies in the fact that the contrast medium concentration, and hence the amount of contrast medium used, may be reduced by as much as a half, as FREYSCHMIDT was able to demonstrate effectively in his experimental study. The scope of angiotomography for improving the diagnosis of angiomas has not yet been fully explored, although - as our experience shows - there may be possibilities.

It is asked, and quite rightly, whether the large number of injections, and hence the amount of contrast medium, does not contribute an additional hazard to the patient. The use of the above-mentioned methods requires no more than about 60 - 70 ml of contrast medium assuming that a part of the radiographic series can be carried out simultaneously or alternately in 2 planes. The use of the less neurotoxic contrast media of the methylglucamine series and the haemodynamic conditions of the angioma show that even larger amount of contrast medium does not involve any greater hazard for patients with arteriovenous angiomas.

It has been the aim of this paper to demonstrate - and I trust that I
have succeeded in doing so - that the further development of angiographic techniques has already contributed towards bringing about a widening of the indications for operation in arteriovenous malformations of
the brain.

Summary

Arteriovenous Angiomas of the Basal Ganglia and Posterior Fossa have
been studied by modern angiographic techniques: Angiocinematography,
Angiotomography and magnification Techniques. The demonstration of the
feeding arteries and drainage veins are even better than with serial-
angiography, and this helps in the decision whether to operate or not.
These are significant developments in the angiographic diagnosis of
angiomas.

References

1. ALLCOCK, J. M.: Angio-Tomography: the technique and its applica-
    tion in investigation of patients with subarachnoid haemorrhage.
    IX Symposium Neuroradiol Göteborg 1970.

2. DECKER, K., BACKMUND: Angiographie des Hirnkreislaufes. Stutt-
    gart: Thieme 1968.

3. DECKER, K., KUNKEL, B.: Zerebrale Angiographie und Hirntod. Fort-
    schr. Röntgenstr. 118, 617-623 (1973).

4. DÜNISCH, O., PFEILER, H., KUHN, H.: Probleme und Aspekte der ra-
    diologischen Vergrösserungstechnik. Electromedica 3, 2-8 (1971).

5. FEKAS, L., GERSTENBRAND, F., KLAUSBERGER, E. M.: Arteriovenöses
    Aneurysma mit Hirnatrophie. Neue Gesichtspunkte bei Verwendung
    des Bewegungsfilmes. Wien. Medizin. Wschr. 109, 61-63 (1959).

6. FREYSCHMIDT, J.: Experimentelle Untersuchungen und Modellversuche
    zur Angiotomographie am Beispiel des thorakolumbalen Spinalarte-
    rienbereiches. Hannover: Habilitationsschrift 1973.

7. GADO, M., BULL, J. W. D.: The carotid angiogram in suprasellar
    masses. Neuroradiology 2, 136-153 (1971).

8. GERHARDT, P., OLDENKOTT, P.: Ergebnisse der Schichtangiographie
    der hinteren Schädelgrube. Acta radiol. (Stockh.) 13, 94-96 (1972).

9. HACKER, H.: Detailangiographie - die direkte Röntgenvergrösserung
    bei der Serienangiographie. Electromedica 6, 346-349 (1970).

10. HALE, J., MISHKIN, M. M.: Serial direct magnification cerebral
    angiography. Amer. J. Roentgenol. 107, 616-620 (1969).

11. KLAUSBERGER, E. M.: Erweiterte Beurteilungsmöglichkeiten bei der
    Angiographie der Hirngefäße. Z. Nervenheilk. (Wien) 20, 108-118
    (1962).

12. NADJMI, M., PÖSCHMANN, H.: Angiotomographie am Diagnost-N. Radiologe 12, 437-440 (1972).

13. OLDENKOTT, P., GERHARDT, P.: Angio-tomography of the posterior fossa. Neuroradiology 2, 212-215 (1971).

14. PIEPGRAS, U., PAMPUS, F., HEUCK, F.: Der Wert der simultanen Angiotomographie für die Diagnostik der Hirngefässaneurysmen. Fortschr. Röntgenstr. 108, 170-176 (1968).

15. PIEPGRAS, U., KAMMERER, V.: Die zerebrale Angiotomographie. Radiologe 12, 431-436 (1972).

16. ROSA, M.: Value of Angio-Tomography in Planning Operative Treatment of Internal Carotid Artery Aneuryms. Neuroradiology 3, 82-91 (1971).

17. WENDE, S., SCHINDLER, K., MORITZ, G.: Der diagnostische Wert der angiographischen Vergrösserungstechnik mit Feinstfokusröhren in zwei Ebenen. Radiologe 11, 471-475 (1971).

18. WAPPENSCHMIDT, J.: Angiotomographische Untersuchungen bei Gefässprozessen. Neuroradiol Symposium. Würzburg 1970.

19. WAPPENSCHMIDT, J., GROTE, W., HOLBACH, K.-H.: Angiographische Befunde vor und nach operativer Behandlung von Gefässmissbildungen des Vertebraliskreislaufes. Acta neurochir. (Wien) 17, 254-273 (1967).

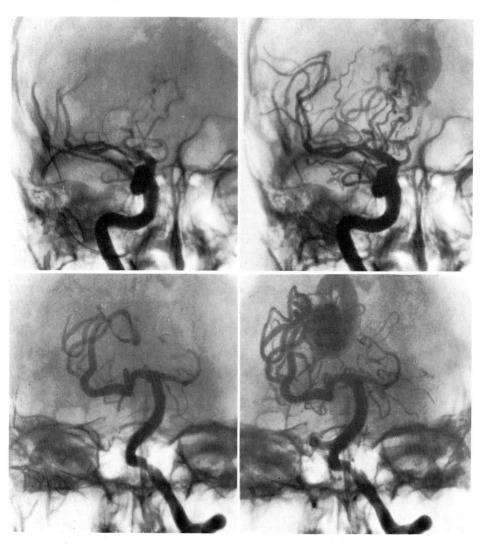

Fig. 1. Angioma of the right basal ganglia. Rapid serial angiography. Good demonstration of the feeding arteries (lenticulostriate A. and branches of posterior cerebral A.) Localisation and angiography enough for judgment "inoperable" angioma

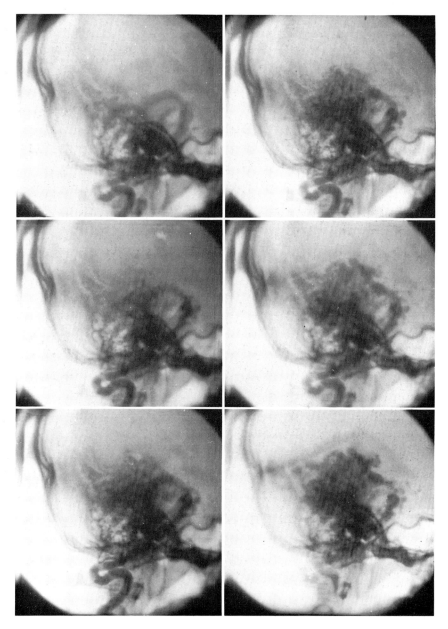

Fig. 2. Angioma in the midline of posterior fossa. Angiocinematography
(70 mm film; 3/sec.) Very good picture size and contrast quality with
demonstration of the feeding A

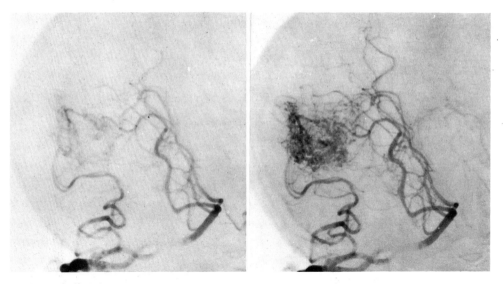

Fig. 3. Angioma in the posterior fossa, right side. Magnification technique (1:2). The feeding aa. can be well judged and differentiated

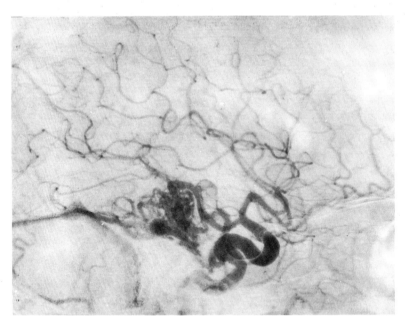

Fig. 4. Angioma left hemisphere, temporo-median. Feeding A. are branches of the posterior cerebral A. Combination with an arterial aneurysm of the posterior cerebral A. Magnification techniques (1:2). Excellent demonstration of the feeding A. and draining veins including the aneurysm

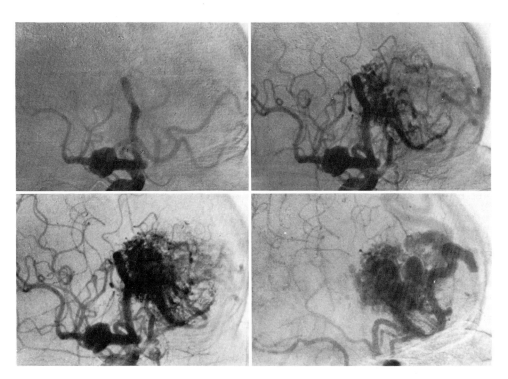

Fig. 5. Angioma of the frontal region combined with an arterial aneurysm of the middle cerebral A. Magnification technique (1:2). Feeding A. are branches of the anterior and middle cerebral A

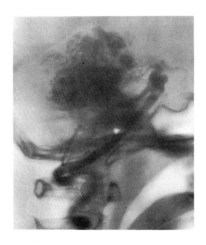

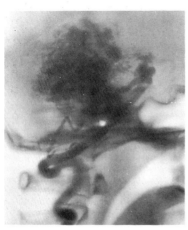

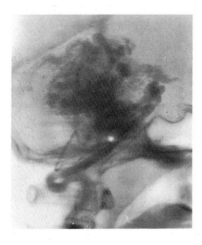

Fig. 6. Same Pat. as Fig. 2. Angiotomography demonstrates the feeding A. and draining veins exactly and better than the other techniques

Superselective Arteriography of the Branches of the External Carotid Artery

R. Djindjian

Selective arteriography of the external and internal carotid branches was an important contribution to neurological angiography. Investigation of the territories of both the internal and external carotid artery can be improved by superselective opacification of their individual branches. Techniques used at present for the external carotid artery are unsuitable for the investigation of the internal carotid. Although opacification of the branches of the external carotid artery has been used previously, it has never been investigated systematically. Since 1970 we have been making a study of this technique, and the following is the report of our results.

Technique

As injection of the contrast medium into the external carotid artery is painful, the investigation is performed under general anesthesia or neurolepto-analgesia. It is also desirable in order to obtain subtraction pictures of high quality.

There are three methods of approach: femoral artery, carotid artery, and superficial temporal artery.

1. Femoral Artery Approach

For many reasons the approach of choice for us is the femoral artery. It allows at the same time investigation of other arteries arising from the aortic arch. Furthermore, an approach from a distance is wise particularly when investigating an angiomatous lesion. This method rarely results in failure, and finally it enables the procedure to be performed with maximum comfort and minimum risk to the radiologist. We used a no. 160 catheter. The tip of the catheter is tapered and slightly curved. Investigation of the left common carotid artery may require a greater curvature of the catheter tip.

2. Carotid Artery Approach

Direct approach to the carotid artery seemed to be the most logical for superselective arteriography, and in fact the first selective arteriographies were done this way (LIVERUND 1958, SCHECHTER 1963, NEWTON,

WEIDNER, and HANAFEE 1966). To us, its advantages were outweighed by its disadvantages, and therefore we preferred the femoral approach.

a) Advantages

Nowadays carotid angiography is a routine investigation: therefore it seemed sensible to use the same puncture for superselective studies.

The carotid approach is the only one possible when the femoral approach is not practicable or when the external carotid artery has been previously ligated. Finally, when placed in the internal carotid artery the catheter can be advanced as far as the cavernous and supracavernous portions of the artery.

b) Disadvantages

However, in practice there are the following disadvantages: Puncture through the soft tissue of the neck hinders the manipulation of the catheter, puncture too close to the bifurcation makes catheterisation difficult. There is some risk in this route of approach and the external carotid artery overlies the proximal collateral branches. Finally, the field of manipulation is small and close to the lesion under investigation.

c) Material Employed

We use a cannula through which a catheter can be inserted. The artery is punctured with a 7 cm long bevelled cannula and stylet. Preliminary injection establishes the situation of the carotid bifurcation and the origin of the main branches of the external carotid artery.

A 30 cm long polyethylene catheter can be introduced with the aid of a no. 105 metallic guide. The catheter itself is very pliable, but if wished, it can be rendered more rigid by using the metallic guide, so making catheterisation more precise.

3. Approach via the Temporal Superficial Artery

The portion of the artery superficial to the temporal fascia and above the parotid gland is exposed or punctured so that a fine catheter can be introduced and passed into the external carotid artery at its origin. This method permits semiselective arteriography, with the tip of the catheter being placed opposite the ostia of the branches of the external carotid artery. It is the least preferred of the three methods, except under the following circumstances:
1. Prolonged catheterisation, as intraarterial chemotherapy.
2. When the external carotid artery has been ligated at its origin.

Method of Examination

1. Superselective arteriography requires initially the visualization of the carotid bifurcation and the branches of the external carotid artery on an X-ray picture or video-tape record (preferably with direct electronic subtraction).

2. After locating the ostia of the branches of the external carotid artery, the tip of the catheter is directed forward or backward according to the branch under examination and then inserted into that

ostium. Collateral branches always rise from the same aspects of the external carotid artery: the superficial temporal, lingual, and facial arteries from the anterior aspect, and the ascending pharyngeal, occipital, and posterior auricular arteries from the posterior aspect. There are variations in the level of origin of each artery, either proximally or distally, and in those on the posterior aspect in the order of origin from the external carotid artery. Providing this has already been established, this does not affect the catheterisation.

The external carotid artery divides in the region of the parotid gland into two branches: its continuation upwards as the superficial temporal artery and the second running obliquely forward as the internal maxillary artery. The tortuosities of the termination of the external carotid artery sometimes make separate injection of the above mentioned branches difficult.

3. Within our experience we have found two causes of failure:

a) marked tortuosity particularly of the terminal part of the external carotid artery;

b) very fine calibre of the branch under investigation; this concerns particularly the posterior auricular and the ascending pharyngeal arteries, if they are not pathologically dilated.

R e s u l t s

Superselective arteriography of the branches of the external carotid artery permits on the one hand isolated opacification of the required area and on the other hand an incomparable concentration of the contrast medium within the most distal branches of each artery. These two features determine the use of this technique in anatomical and hemodynamic studies as well as for diagnostic and therapeutic purposes.

I. A n a t o m y

These selective injections enabled us to analyse the cervico-cephalic vascular tree and each of its territories during the three phases of angiography . We were able to demonstrate the character and the importance of the anastomosis between different branches of the external carotid artery as well as the anastomosis with the opposite side and with the internal carotid and subclavian vessels. Finally we were able to define the blood supply of the soft tissues and mucosa and to demonstrate the venous drainage of each of the territories concerned.

1. Selective catheterisation of different branches of the external carotid artery.

The variations in origin do not hinder the selective study of these vessels. Although they may have different levels of origin in relation to the carotid bifurcation or may originate from a common trunk, they always originate from the same aspect of the external carotid artery so that it is almost always possible to perform selective arteriography of the common trunk.

The first and the most simple to catheterise is the superior thyroid artery which is the first anterior branch and is situated immediately above the bifurcation or at the bifurcation of the common carotid.

The lingual artery (Fig. 1) and the facial artery (Figs. 2, 3) also originate from the anterior aspect of the external carotid, sometimes from a common trunk, together with the superior thyroid artery.

On turning the tip of the catheter posteriorly one usually finds the ostium of the occipital artery (Fig. 4). However, its position is variable and may be located anywhere between the bifurcation and the termination of the external carotid artery.

On the posterior aspect of the external carotid, the ascending pharyngeal artery (Fig. 5) has a constant origin and is followed by the posterior auricular artery (Fig. 6) (sometimes the sequence is reversed). They are narrow and more difficult to catheterise unless they become dilated due to the pathological processes taking place in the territory of their supply.

The terminal part of the external carotid can be catheterised in the majority of cases.
The superficial temporal artery (Fig. 7) is the continuation of the external carotid and is easily accessible. In certain cases it is even possible to catheterise one of its external branches: the frontal or parietal artery.

The internal maxillary artery (Fig. 8) is found opposite the condyle of the mandible. The tip of the catheter is directed anteriorly and at that level points towards the ostium of the artery. Sometimes it is possible to perform superselective arteriography of the middle meningeal artery (Fig. 9).

II. D i a g n o s i s

The independent demonstration of each of the areas supplied by branches of the external carotid artery allows more exact localisation and definition of the arterial feeders. Above all, this technique enables opacification of the lesions, which were previously arteriographically avascular. Telangiectasias, capillary angiomas, venous and cavernous angiomas, and bony lesions of different types can be opacified. There is no tendency for the blood to flow preferentially into these lesions; on the contrary, the fine net of afferent arterioles constitutes a kind of a barrier. Superselective arteriography enables these lesions to be differentiated from truly avascular ones.

III. I n d i c a t i o n s   f o r   T r e a t m e n t

One of the greatest advantages of superselective arteriography has been to open to the angioradiologist the vast field of therapy.

Superselective arteriography permits embolisation (with GELFOAM - Fig. 10) through the catheter to be performed with good results. The main indication is the treatment of arteriovenous fistulae, but it can also be used for other arteriovenous malformations. Good results have also been obtained in the prevention of hemorrhage and lessening of the dystrophy which occurs in soft tissues in contact with the angioma has been noted. These results suggest that this type of embolisation is the treatment of choice. The superiority embolisation over a ligature

is obvious, as it permits distal closure of a vessel while preserving
the patency of proximal parts of the artery so that this can be used
again in case the malformation refills through collaterals.

Another field of application is the preoperative occlusion of arteries
supplying a tumor. Considerable reduction in the bulk of the tumor may
be achieved, if such lesions as meningiomas, glomus tumors, nasopharyn-
geal fibromas etc. are embolised before the attempted excision.

Finally superselective arteriography has a wide application in the
treatment of malignant diseases of the head and neck. The technique
has the following advantages:

Firstly, apart from supplying topographical data, it allows one to determine whether the lesion is hyper- or hypovascular, and in this way
one may predict the efficacy of eventual chemotherapy

Secondly, the reduction of the bulk of the tumor, which may be achieved
through embolisation, will probably form part of the management of the
tumor either as a preliminary to surgery or as a supplement to radiotherapy or chemotherapy.

There is no doubt that what has been achieved by selective arteriography
of the external carotid and by medullary angiography could in future
be attempted in selective internal carotid angiography (Fig.11) and in
visceral arteriography, thus adding promising new dimensions to the
treatment of such conditions as respiratory tract, gastro-intestinal,
and renal hemorrhages.

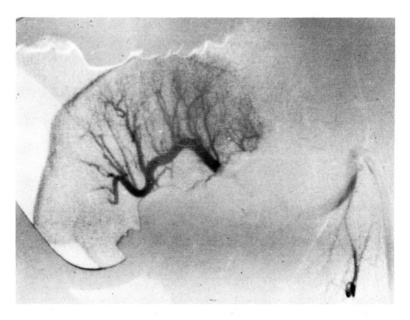

Fig. 1. Superselective arteriography of the lingual artery via the
femoral route

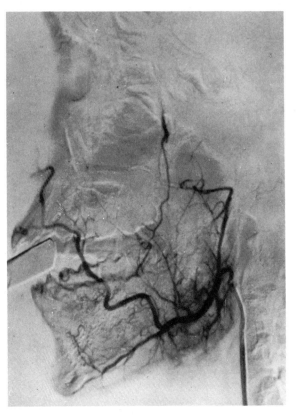

Fig. 2. Superselective
arteriography of the
facial artery via the
femoral route

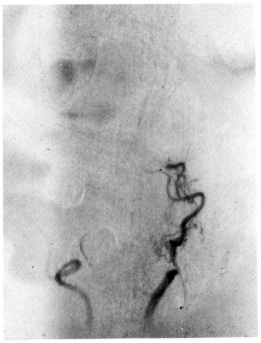

Fig. 3. Superselective
arteriography of the
arteria palatina as-
cendens via the femor-
al route

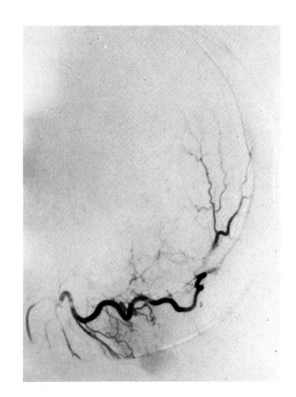

Fig. 4. Superselective arteriography of the occipital artery via the femoral route

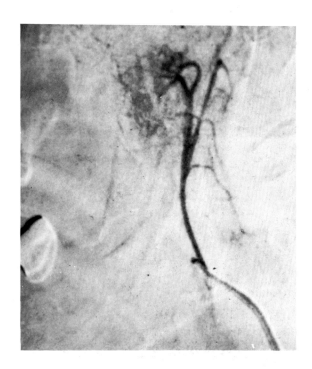

Fig. 5. Superselective arteriography of the ascending pharyngeal artery via the femoral route

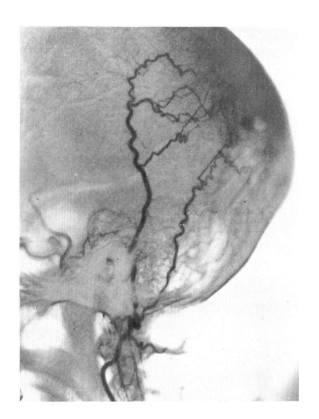

Fig. 6. Superselective arteriography of the posterior auricular artery via the femoral route

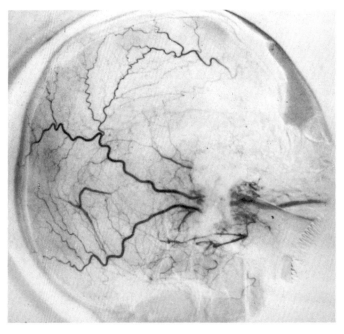

Fig. 7. Superselective arteriography of the superficial temporal artery via the femoral route

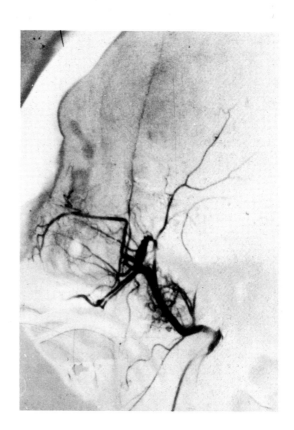

Fig. 8. Superselective arteriography of the internal maxillary artery via the femoral route

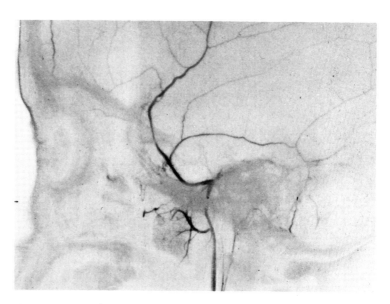

Fig. 9. Superselective arteriography of the middle meningeal artery via the femoral route

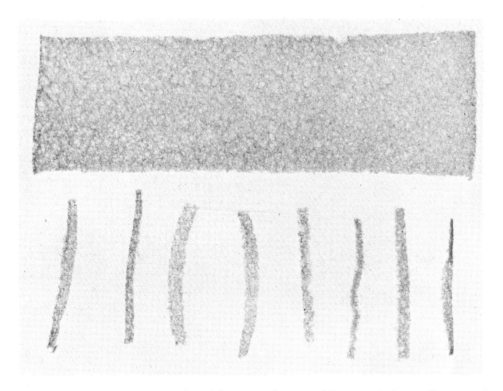

Fig. 10. Above: strips of gelfoam. Below: Gelfoam cut into fine strips ready to be injected

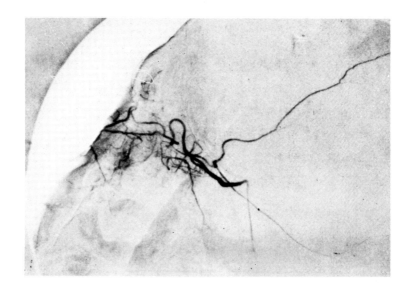

Fig. 11. Superselective arteriography of the ophthalmic artery using the cervical route

Use of Intraoperative Angiography

F. PEETERS

Introduction

Two methods of introducing contrast agents into the cerebral vessels in angiography are available today.

The simplest method in carotid angiography is direct percutaneous puncture of the carotid artery. Catheterisation, either from the brachial artery or from the femoral artery, is usually preferred in vertebral angiography. Direct puncture of the vertebral artery has recently been advocated again (1).

Catheterisation of the desired blood vessel from the femoral artery is the method of choice in intraoperative angiography both of the carotid and vertebral arteries. The catheter may be left in situ throughout the operation and angiography will in no way interfere with surgery as the site of introduction is situated far from the operative field.

Intraoperative angiography has so far only been carried out on a restricted scale, although the procedure has been used since 1966 (2) on the carotid during the surgical treatment of aneurysms as well as angiomas. Only a single case of intraoperative vertebral angiography was found to have been reported in the literature (3).

The quality of the angiograms will vary with the radiological equipment available in the operating room. The results obtained with the most simple apparatus will suffice when angiography is designed to check the extent to which an angioma has been removed, the clipping of an aneurysm or the relative positions of a probe and an angioma.

The last-named procedure is of importance in cryosurgery for the treatment of arteriovenous malformations. Lesions which are inoperable because of their deep-seated location and the dangers of the approach may be reached by the cryoprobe without exposing the vascular malformation. The relative positions of the probe and the malformation are checked by intraoperative angiography.

Material and Methods

Since 1969, intraoperative carotid angiography has been carried out by the present author in fifteen patients. In thirteen cases, the procedure was used to localize the cryoprobe in the cryosurgery of angiomas which were inoperable by other methods. In one case, the clipping of vessels supplying an angioma was checked.

Intraoperative vertebral angiography was carried out in five cases. In three cases, this was done to determine the relative positions of the cryoprobe and of angiomas located in the thalamus, which were solely supplied by branches of the homolateral posterior cerebral artery. In two cases, angiography was carried out to check the effect of ligation of afferent vessels to deep-seated angiomas which were solely supplied by branches of the basilar artery.

Despite the drawback of the catheter remaining in the blood stream for 3-4 hours in every case, the only possible complication observed in one of the patients following intraoperative carotid angiography consisted of a minor pulmonary embolus which appeared within a few days of the operation; no further complications occurred.

Catheterisation is carried out from one of the two femoral arteries following insertion of the catheter by Seldinger's technique.

The measurements of the catheters are as follows: carotid artery: inner diameter 1.20 mm., outer diameter 2.20 mm.; vertrebral artery: inner diameter 1.14 mm., outer diameter 1.65 mm.

A total quantity of 100 - 150 ml. of contrast medium is injected during operation, 10 ml. being administered per injection.

The considerable length of time required for the operation in cryosurgery is due, among other things, to the fact that, depending on the size of the lesion, freezing is essential at numerous sites within the malformation. Initially, the cryoprobe was introduced into the malformation in several directions through a single opening in the dura mater. The direction was controlled by the intraoperative angiograms. Fig. 1 shows the probe located within the malformation, anteroposterior view. The various positions of the probe during freezing are drawn in the first X-ray so that the points at which the probe was situated can ultimately be seen in the angiogram. Fig. 2 shows a similar situation; lateral view.

The quality of the X-rays taken during intraoperative vertebral angiography is approximately identical with that of the X-rays taken in carotid angiography (Fig. 3). In some cases, the laborious operation of correctly introducing the probe may be shortened by using a measuring system making it possible to decide in advance at which points the probe will enter the malformation. For this purpose, a perforated perspex disc was used, the diameters of the perforations being such as to allow the probe to pass exactly through them. The perforations are spaced 0.5 cm. apart. The disc is fixed to the trephine hole by three bolts. It can be established from the X-ray (Fig. 4) into which holes the probe has to be inserted to reach the entire malformation. In addition, the depth can be determined from the anteroposterior angiogram. The drawback to this procedure is that puncture tracks diverging from a single puncture are not produced but that parallel tracks are formed from a number of punctures. On the other hand, this method does make possible an even distribution of the frozen areas throughout the angioma.

The full benefit of cryosurgery can be derived by introducing the cryoprobe into the malformation through a drill hole using a stereotaxic apparatus. A condition is that the stereotaxic apparatus can be used to locate the lesion and that the malformation is a small one. The present author has been able so far to use the stereotaxic apparatus for this purpose on two occasions. It is possible in principle to make a stereotaxic apparatus suitable for all locations.

The question of whether ligation of afferent vessels is a suitable method for the treatment of angiomas is beyond the scope of the present paper. When it is decided to use this method of treatment, intraoperative angiography may be useful both in making sure that the right vessels are clipped and to gain an immediate impression of the effect of ligation. Figs. 5 and 6 show an instance in which an angioma initially appeared to be supplied by three branches of the left posterior cerebral artery. It is true that, when the first clips were applied, a considerable part of the lesion was no longer filled with contrast material, but a new afferent branch arising from the posterior communication artery was then visualized.

C o m m e n t

Although this is not supported by the findings reported in the literature (4), vertebral angiography has a worse reputation than carotid angiography as far as appearance of complications is concerned. The proportion of neurological complications varies from 0.2 to 0.5 percent in the two procedures. Moreover, it is pointed out that the complication rate in vertebral angiography is not related either to the number of injections or to the total volume of contrast medium injected.

The haemodynamic equilibrium is more likely to be upset in catheterisation of the vertebral artery than it is in catheterisation of the carotid artery. Apart from the smaller diameter of the vertebral artery, the flow of blood through this vessel may be affected to a greater extent by the position of the head than is that through the carotid artery. In five out of fourty-one subjects, extension and rotation of the head were found to result in total occlusion of the vertebral artery on the side away from which the head had been rotated (5).

The circulation in the contralateral vertebral artery may be completely interrupted both on extension and on rotation of the head (6). Fig. 7 shows an instance of local constriction of the left vertebral artery on rotation of the head to the right. When the head is in the neutral position, the left vertebral artery will permit an adequate flow of blood.

In view of the above, the head should be in a neutral position in intraoperative vertebral angiography. Extension and rotation should be avoided.

Despite the considerable length of time required for catheterisation and the large volume of contrast medium administered, intraoperative angiography of the carotid as well as of the vertebral artery may be regarded as a safe neuroradiological aid in the neurosurgical treatment of angiomas.

S u m m a r y

A report is made on the use of carotid and vertebral angiography during the surgical treatment of angiomas which cannot be excised because
of their location and extent.

In cryosurgery, angiography is designed to check the relative positions
of the cryoprobe and the malformation. When afferent vessels are ligated, the effect of occlusion of the vessels can be directly assessed.

Intraoperative angiography was found to be a safe procedure.

R e f e r e n c e s

1. RUGGIERO, G., SCIALFA, G., CRISTI, G.: The value of direct percutaneous puncture technique in vertebral angiography. Neuroradiology 6, 104-109 (1973).

2. LOOP, J. W., FOLTZ, E. L.: Applications of angiography during intracranial operation. Acta radiol. (Diagn.) 5, 363-367 (1966).

3. DRAKE, C. G.: Further experience with surgical treatment of aneurysms of the basilar artery. J. Neurosurg. 29, 372-392 (1968).

4. WISHART, D. L. Complications in vertebral angiography as compared
   to non-vertebral cerebral angiography in 447 studies. Amer. J.
   Roentgenol. 113, 527-537 (1971).

5. BROWN, B. St. J., TISSINGTON TATLOW, W. F.: Radiographic studies
   of the vertebral arteries in cadavers. Radiology 81, 80-88 (1963).

6. TIWISINA, T.: Die Vertebralis-Angiographie. Heidelberg: Hüthig
   1964.

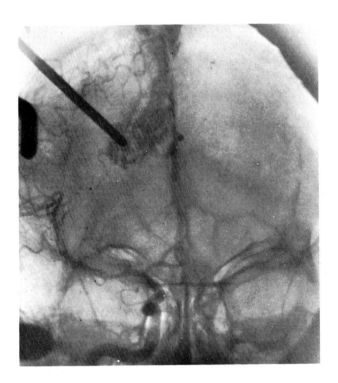

Fig. 1. Intraoperative right carotid angiogram, anteroposterior view. The cryoprobe is situated within the angioma

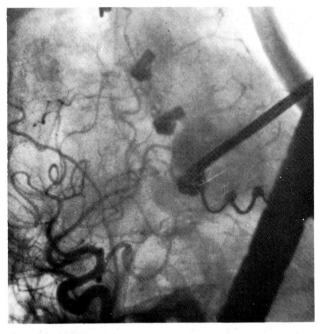

Fig. 2. Intraoperative right carotid angiogram, lateral view. The cryoprobe in situ in the angioma. Previous positions of the cryoprobe within the angioma have been drawn in the angiogram

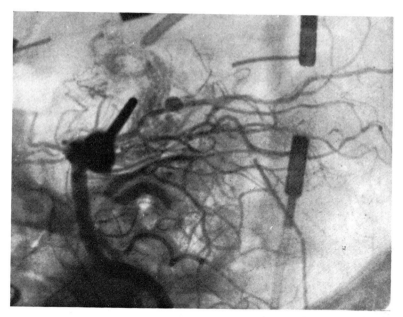

Fig. 3. Intraoperative left carotid angiogram, lateral view. A perspex disc perforated with holes 0.5 cm. apart has been fixed to the trephine hole. The cryoprobe has been introduced into the angioma through one of the perforations

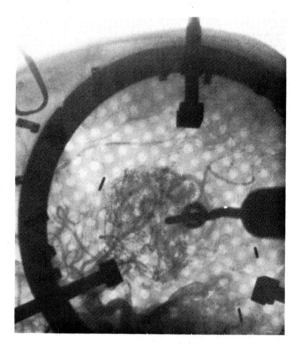

Fig. 4. Intraoperative left vertebral angiogram, lateral view. The cryoprobe is situated close to the malformation

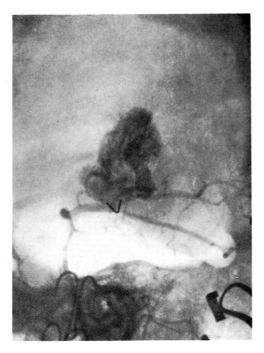

Fig. 5. Intraoperative left vertebral angiogram, lateral view. Open
clip for localization of afferent artery which is to be clipped

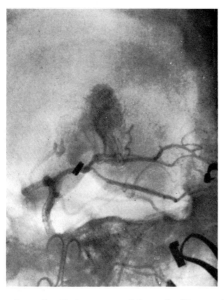

Fig. 6. Intraoperative left vertebral angiogram, lateral view. Same
patient as in Fig. 5, after occlusion of one of the afferent vessels.
Increased filling of posterior communicating artery

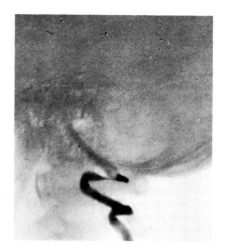

Fig. 7. Left vertebral angiogram, lateral view. Occlusion of left vertebral artery by rotation of head to the right

Extracranial and Extra-Intracranial Arteriovenous Angiomas

A. L. AGNOLI

Introduction

Improvements in neurosurgical technique, particularly microsurgery and
embolization, have widened the operative possibilities, not only for
intracerebral, but also for extracerebral vascular malformations.

The aim of the neuroradiologist is to reveal the chief hemodynamic aspects of these malformations, i.e. to demonstrate all supplying and
draining vessels, the localization and extent of the malformation,
and to demonstrate the intracranial and intradural part of the angioma.
The classification of TÖNNIS (101) based on VIRCHOW, as well as the
classifications of OLIVECRONA and collaborators (75), KRAYENBÜHL and
collaborators (49), MCCORMICK (64), and AMICO and collaborators (1)
are only of anatomico-pathological importance, and are not suitable
in practice for judging the operability of the lesion. A simple classification based on the localization seems also unsatisfactory, but is
necessary for a general review.

Our material comprises 21 patients with extracranial and extra-intra-
cranial arteriovenous angiomas. We have had the opportunity of analys-
ing 3 further cases thanks to the courtesy of KOHLMEYER of the Department of Neurology, Giessen.

Material

Arteriovenous Angiomas in the Orbits

7 patients had arteriovenous angiomas localized to the orbits and adjacent soft tissues (Table 1).

The main symptoms were exophthalmus, a bruit synchronous with the pulse,
and diminished movement of the eye-ball. One patient had weakness of
the sixth nerve and ipsilateral increase of the deep tendon reflexes.
One patient suffered from repeated bleeding from the angioma, and 4
patients complained of orbital pain. Routine X-rays were normal in all
patients except one, in whom widening of the superior orbital fissure
was found.

We were able to distinguish two types of malformation:

The first type is supplied by the ophthalmic artery (48). It drains
through the superior ophthalmic vein into the cavernous sinus. The
drainage takes place quite rapidly, within 4 seconds.

Table 1. Orbital - Angiomas

Patient Case hist. No.	History	Arterial supply	Operation
1. G. A. m, 46y 527/57	6 mths.	A. maxillaris int. A. ophthalmica	Ext. and int. carotid ligation. Recurrence
2. B. R. f, 2y 2621/60	since birth	Left A. ophthalmica	None
3. B. F. m, 61 y 680/63	40 yrs.	Right A. ophthalmica and left A. angularis	2 x ligation. Excision. No recurrence
4. K. H. m, 25 y 352/65	5 yrs.	A. ophthalmica and left A. maxillaris	3 x ligation. Excision. No recurrence
5. P. C. f, 4 y 422/68	since birth	A. temporalis superf., A. angularis Mandibularis, dilated A. ophthalmica	None. Radiation therapy
6. G. M. f, 1 y 509/69	few months	A. ophthalmica	Ext. and int. carotid ligation. Cardiac arrest
7. F. R. m, 2 y 377/71	since birth	Right A. ophthalmica and right A. facialis	Total excision. No recurrence.

67

The second type is supplied by the ophthalmic artery and internal maxillary artery (15, 20, 60, 108). Feeding vessels from the vertebral and superior thyroid artery have also been observed (95). Such malformations are localized not only within the orbits, but extend into the adjacent soft tissues of the face. Venous drainage is often delayed. In one patient the pathologically widened draining veins were seen 8 seconds after the injection of the contrast medium. We have performed orbital phlebography in three patients. In none of them was the angioma demonstrated.

Arteriovenous Angiomas of the Face

This group comprises 8 patients (Table 2).

Feeding vessels can be demonstrated by selective (41, 96) (Fig. 1) and superselective (23, 24, 25) angiography.

The main symptoms were a bruit synchronous with the pulse, local tenderness in 2 patients, headaches in 2 patients, and recurrent bleeding from the buccal mucosa and loss of teeth in 3 patients. One patient had mental symptoms, and another slight exaggeration of the ipsilateral tendon reflexes.

Plain X-rays revealed thinning of the bone texture corresponding to the site of the malformation in two patients. Malformations drained through the veins of the galea, the facial veins, and the jugular veins though at a slightly slower rate than is seen in cases of intracerebral angiomas (41). These malformations are sometimes supplied by a single artery (36, 41, 95, 108, 111) originating from the external carotid artery, most frequently via the superficial temporal artery. The latter is most frequently the vessel of supply in traumatic arteriovenous fistulae and aneurysms (4, 15, 51, 78, 89).

Arteriovenous angiomas supplied by all branches of the external carotid artery constitute a considerable diagnostic and therapeutic problem (62). Such patients often have fatal hemorrhage after an attempt at tooth extraction (37, 58, 84). A similar case is personally known to us*. Such bleeding can sometimes be stopped only by a radical procedure including the resection of the mandible (61).

Case Report

A 12-year-old girl had had since birth an extensive angioma of the left side of the face, and there had been several episodes of transient senso-motor weakness of the right extremities. Plan X-rays showed asymmetry of the skull with increased density of the base and asymmetry of the petrous pyramids. Air encephalography revealed an asymmetry of the ventricular system. Left sided carotid angiography showed that the malformation (Fig. 2) was supplied by all branches of the external carotid artery. As far as the intracerebral circulation was concerned, only the territory of the Sylvian artery filled with the contrast medium (Fig. 3). Ligation of the external carotid artery was unsuccessful, and the postoperative angiogram showed that the malformation was supplied by the anastomoses from the left internal carotid and ophthal-

---

* F. HERGET, Department of Anesthesiology, Center of Surgery, University of Giessen

Table 2. Angiomas in the face

Patient Case hist. No.	History	Arterial supply	Operation
1. B. H. m, 22 y 3179/58	6 months	Both Aa. temp. superficialis, left Occ. externa	Ligation and excision. No recurrence
2. B. G. m, 35 y 3269/60	15 years	Thyroidea cranialis, A. facialis	3 x ligation without effect
3. H. M. f, 35 y 393/67	2 years	Temporalis superficialis, Occipitalis	Ligation. Total excision. No recurrence.
4. H. E. f, 25 y 804/70	few months	Temporalis superficialis	Total excision. No recurrence.
5. T. I. m, 22 y 882/70	3 years	Temporalis superficialis, Occipitalis externa	Total excision. No recurrence.
6. A. D. f, 67 y 89/71	2 years	Temporalis superficialis, left A. auricularis	Ligation. No recurrence.
7. M. A. m, 13 y 432/72	many yrs.	External carotid circulation, branches of A. vertebralis	Ligation of Carotis ext., No effect.
8. B. R. m, 10 y 31/73	2 years	A. carotis externa	Ligation of Carotis ext., No effect.

69

mic arteries (Fig. 4). Other feeding vessels originated from the right vertebral and occipital arteries as well as from the dilated right ophthalmic artery, which was supplied directly from the posterior communicating artery (Fig. 5).

The intracerebral vessels of the left side were not demonstrated, probably due to the existing steal. The left internal carotid artery seemed to be occluded at the level of the siphon.

Occipito-Cervical Angiomas (Table 3)

It is well known that traumatic arteriovenous fistulae occur in this region more frequently than do congenital angiomas (9, 28, 59, 92). The vertebral artery is surrounded by well-developed venous channels (50). This favors the occurrence of arteriovenous fistulae, which may be a complication of angiography (6, 68). The malformation may be supplied by the vertebral artery only (27, 35, 49, 73, 82, 102) or by the vertebral artery and the thyro-cervical trunk (22 , 33, 46, 54, 96, 97). Other vessels of supply include the contralateral vertebral artery (12, 53, 80, 88) and the contralateral occipital artery (3, 12, 36, 47 , 55, 62, 83, 87, 95, 111). The main symptom in this group of angiomas is the bruit synchronous with the pulse. Neurological signs suggest an intracranial or intraspinal extension of the malformation. PYGOTT et al. (80) reported in 1964 a patient with an occipito-cervical angioma and a tetraparesis probably due to ischemia of the spinal cord. A case with extraspinal extension of the occipito-cervical angioma and recurrent subarachnoid hemorrhage is reported by ZIERSKI. Intracranial extension of these malformations has been rarely reported (12, 49, 50, 87, 108). We had the opportunity of observing such a patient in whom angiography demonstrated an occipito-cervical angioma with intracranial extension (Figs. 6 and 7). The malformation drained to the transverse and sigmoid sinuses. The patient died because of myocardial infarct, and autopsy confirmed the intracranial dural extension of the angioma.

Direct communication between the external carotid artery and a venous sinus:

Cases with direct communication between the branches of the external carotid artery and intracranial sinuses have been reported in the literature. These malformations constitute a particular neuroradiological problem. The communication can sometimes be missed because of the rapid filling of the jugular vein (50). A pathologically enlarged occipital artery may run directly into the transverse sinus (32, 36, 69, 87, 83), the sigmoid sinus (100, 109) or other dural sinuses (11, 65, 66, 81). Direct communication between branches of the external carotid artery and the external jugular vein, not arising after trauma has also been reported (62, 78, 98, 107). NICOLA et al. (72) reported in 1968 a case of fistula between the external occipital artery and the transverse sinus accompanied by neurological deficits. A similar case was under our care. Angiography showed an abnormal origin of the dilated occipital and lingual arteries from the carotid bifurcation. The occipital artery drained directly into the transverse and sigmoid sinuses.

Dural Arteriovenous Angiomas

Arteriovenous malformations involving the dura are mostly localized to the posterior fossa. They are supplied either from the meningeal branches of the external carotid artery (13, 29, 65, 70, 72, 76, 105, 106)

Table 3. Occipito - cervical angiomas

Patient Case hist. No.	History	Arterial supply	Operation
1. S. I. f, 45 y 424/67	many years	Occ. externa, Thyreo-cervicalis Vertebralis	Several times ligation. Recurrence.
2. Ü. L. f, 50 y 307/69	1 year	Occ. ext., both vertebral arteries Thyreo-cervicalis, cerebellar artery	Extirpation. Exitus due to cardiac arrest
3. B. K. m, 6 y 182/70, 631/72	1 year	Occ. ext., Thyreo-cervicalis, both vertebral arteries.	Extirpation. No recurrence.
4. L. H. m, 24 y 656/71	2 years	Left dilated A. occipitalis.	Ligation Exitus due to arterial thrombosis
5. W. R. f, 15 y 537/72, 34/73	6 weeks	A. vertebralis, Thyreo-cervicalis. Occ. ext., radicular arteries.	Incomplete excision.

or the vertebral artery (52, 74). These malformations may also be supplied exclusively from the internal carotid artery (14, 94).

However, in the majority of cases the feeding meningeal branches are
multiple and originate from the external and internal carotid arteries
(17, 26, 45, 50, 63, 70, 91), from the vertebral and internal carotid
arteries (40), or from the external, internal, and vertebral arteries
at the same time (17, 31, 43, 52, 76, 77, 104). Angiomas are only rarely localized to the frontal region (57, 71, 79). We have had the opportunity of observing two patients with such a localization of their
angiomas*.

In our cases the malformation was supplied through the anterior ethmoidal artery and drained through dilated veins (Fig. 8). Selective
angiography of the external carotid artery filled the feeding meningeal branches (Fig. 9).

In both cases the main symptom was subarachnoid hemorrhage.

Discussion

Congenital angiomas develop before the formation of the coverings of the
CNS, i.e. in the third to fourth week of embryonic life (75) and are
due to defects of the capillary system (50, 85). From the second month
of embryonic life the system does not differ from the vascular net of
an adult (36). The late signs and symptoms of these arteriovenous malformations are apparently due to the rupture of arteriovenous septa
(57), which constitute the rest of the primitive short-circuit between
arteries and veins.

The patients seek medical help mainly because of the bruit, for cosmetic
reasons, or because of ill-defined symptoms of pressure within the head
or headache. Neurological signs are encountered mostly in cases of intracranial extension of the angioma. Angiomas involving the mucosa often cause recurrent bleeding or loss of teeth. Sometimes signs of cardiac insufficiency (10, 33, 73, 88) are encountered. The main symptom
which directs attention towards the diagnosis of an arteriovenous malformation is the bruit.

Orbital (34, 103, 110) angiomas or arteriovenous malformations of the
face (38) are less frequent than tumors of these regions, but in relation to intracerebral arteriovenous angiomas their occurrence is
more frequent than the literature would suggest (75, 78). Extracranial
vascular malformations combined with one or more intracerebral arteriovenous malformations are infrequent (2, 15, 16, 19, 21, 41, 50, 54, 67,
78, 99).

Simple ligation of the feeding vessel can be successful only in cases
in which the malformation is supplied by one arterial branch (3, 7, 18,
42, 59, 78, 81, 97, 98, 108, 109, 111). Out of the 75 dural angiomas
reported, 30 patients were not operated upon. 28 patients had a simple
ligation of the supplying vessels. In 18 of them recurrence occurred.
In 7 patients the angioma was operated upon microsurgically and completely excised without recurrence. Complete excision of arteriovenous
angiomas of extracerebral vessels has been postulated in all cases
(12, 29, 36, 47, 59, 73, 90, 95, 111). Simple ligation is unsuccessful
because of the profuse anastomoses (8, 86). Palliative procedures are

---

* Thanks to the courtesy of K. KOHLMEYER, Center of Neurology, University of Giessen

usually followed by recurrence (12, 33, 36, 47, 50, 91, 98, 111). In some cases of traumatic arteriovenous fistulas (30, 90, 92, 95) or fistulas resulting from puncture during angiography (5, 35, 68, 78), natural cures have been reported. Spontaneous cures have also been reported in cases of congenital arteriovenous malformations (16, 44) but they remain exceptional.

Large angiomas of the soft tissues of the face cause considerable difficulties. Ligation of the feeding vessels can increase the steal syndrom and impair the intracranial circulation. It is still too early to judge the late results of embolization technique which has been introduced in recent years into the management of angiomas supplied by extracranial vessels.

R e f e r e n c e s

1. AMICO, G., CANEPARI, C.: Le communicazioni arterio-venose anomale spontane tra carotide externa e seni durali. G. Psichiatr. Neuropathol., 98, 469-491 (1970).

2. ARNULF, G., DUQUESNEI, J.: Anéurisme artério-veineux congenital de la région frontale chez l'enfant. Phlébologie, 21, 357-362 (1968).

3. BARTAL, A. D., LEVY, M. L.: Excision of a congenital suboccipital vertebral arterio-venous fistula. J. Neurosurg. 37, 452-455 (1972).

4. BARTHOLIN: zit. nach SCHECHTER et al. 1971.

5. BERGQUIST, E.:Bilateral arteriovenous fistulae. A complication of vertebral angiography by direct percutaneous puncture: two cases, one with spontaneous closure. Brit. J. Radiol. 44, 519-523 (1971).

6. BERGSTRÖM, K., LODIN, H.: Arteriovenous fistulae as a complication of cerebral angiography, report of three cases. Brit. J. Radiol. 39, 263-266 (1966).

7. BERRY, J.: Large arterio-venous aneurysm of the neck treated by excision. Lancet II, 1714-1716 (1906).

8. BOSNIAK, M. A.: Cervical arterial pathways associated with brachiocephalic occlusive disease. Amer. J. Roentgen. 91, 1232-1244 (1964).

9. CALLANDER, C. L.: Study of arterio-venous fistula with an analysis of 447 cases. Hopkins Hosp. Rep. 19, 259-358 (1920).

10. CAROLL, C. P. H., JAKOBY, R. K.:Neonatal congestive heart failure as the symptom of cerebral arteriovenous malformation. J. Neurosurg. 25, 159-163 (1966).

11. CASTAIGNE, P., LAPLANE, D., DJINDJIAN, R., BORIES, J., AUGUSTIN, P.: Communication artério-veineuse spontanée entre la carotide externe et le sinus caverneux. Rev. Neurol. 5, 114-122 (1965).

12. CHOU, S. N., STORY, J. L., SELJESKOG, F. et al.: Further experience with arteriovenous fistulas of the certebral artery in the neck. Surgery 62, 779-788 (1967).

13. CIMINELLO, V. J., SACHS, E. Jr.: Arteriovenous malformations of the posterior fossa. J. Neurosurg. 19, 602-604 (1962).

14. CORTES, O., CHASE, N. E., LEEDS, N.: Visualization of tentorial branches of internal carotid artery in intracranial lesions other than meningiomas. Radiology 82, 1024-1028 (1964).

15. DANDY, W. E.:Arteriovenous aneurysms of scalp and face. Arch. Surg. 52, 1 (1946).

16. DAVID, M., PRADAT, P., DILENGE, D., DA LAGE, C., MESSIMY, R.: Hémangiome extra-dural temporal associé à une malformation artério-veineuse supérieure d'aspect fugace. Neuro-Chirurgie (Paris) 13, 725-735 (1967).

17. DEBRUN, G., CHARTRES, A.: Infra and supratentorial arteriovenous malformations. A general review. Neuroradiology 3, 184-192 (1972).

18. DEPRÈS, M.: Tumeur veineuse du plancher de la bouche. Anévrysme artérioveineux. Ligature des deux artères linguales. Bull. Soc. Chir. Paris 5, 794-800 (1879).

19. DI CHIRO, G.: Combined retine-cerebellar angiomatosis and deep cervical angiomas, case report. J. Neurosurg. 14, 685-687 (1957).

20. DILENGE, D., FISCHGOLD, H., DAVIS, M.: L'artère ophthalmique aspects angiographiques. Neuro-Chirurgie (Paris) 7, 249-257 (1961).

21. DILENGE, D., DAVID, M., ROESER, J., ABOULKER, A.: Anévrysmes artérioveineux cerébraux par l'angiographic de l'artère carotide externe. Neuro-Chirurgie 9, 365-370 (1963).

22. DJINDJIAN, R.: Angiography of the spinal cord. Baltimore University Park Press. pp. 172-179 (1970).

23. DJINDJIAN, R., MERLAND, J. J., REY, A., THUREL, J., HOUDART, R.: Artériographic super sélective de la carotide externa. Neuro-Chirurgie, 19, 165-171 (1973).

24. DJINDJIAN, R., COPHIGNON, J., REY, A., THÉRON, J., MERLAND, J. J., HOUDART, R.: Superselective arteriographic embolization by the femorale route in neuroradiology. Study of 50 cases. III embolization in craniocerebral pathology. Neuroradiology 6, 143-152 (1973).

25. DJINDJIAN, R., COPHIGNON, J., REY, A., THÉRON, J., MERLAND, J. J., HOUDART, R.: Superselective arteriographic embolization by the femorale route in neuroradiology. Study of 50 cases. II embolization in vertrebromedullary pathology. Neuroradiology 6, 132-142 (1973).

26. DOYON, D., METZGER, J.: Malformations vasculaires isolées sus tentorielles (à l'excision des fistulas carotido-caverneuses). 9e Symposium de Neuroradiologie de Göteborg - 24 au 29 S. 70.

27. EHRLICH, F. E., CAREY, L., KIHINOS, N. S.: Congenital arteriovenous fistula between the vertebral artery and vertebral vein: case report. J. Neurosurg. 29, 629-630 (1968).

28. ELKIN, D. C., HARRIS, M. H.: Arteriovenous aneurysms of vertebral vessels: report of 10 cases. Ann. Surg. 124, 934-951 (1946).

29. FADHLI, M. A.:Congenital arterio-venous fistula involving the occipital artery and lateral venous sinus; case report. J. Neurosurg. 39, 289-300 (1969).

30. FAETH, W. H., DUECKER, H. W.:Arteriovenous vascular malformation of the cervical portion of the vertebral artery; case report. Neurology 11, 492-493 (1961).

31. FRUGONI, P., RUBERTI, R.: Observations sur 54 cas d'anévrysmes artério-veineux sus-tentoriels traités chirugicalement. Neuro-Chirurgie (Paris) 9, 377 - 389 (1963).

32. FUKIYMA, K., NAKASHIMA, Y., NISHIMARU, K., TAKEYA, J., KATSUKI, S.: Idiopathic arterio-venous fistula involving the occipital artery and the transverse venous sinus: a case report. Brain Nerve (Tokyo) 23, 1307-1310 (1971).

33. GERACI, A. R., UPSON, J. F., GREENE, D. G.: Congenital vertebral arteriovenous fistula. JAMA 210, 727-728 (1969).

34. GLONING, K., HAIDEN, K.: Angiographische Diagnose eines orbitalen Tumors. Wien. Z. Nervenheilk., 7, 58 (1953).

35. GOODY, W., SCHECHTER, M.: Congenital cervical arteriomalformations. Brit. J. Radiol. 33, 709-711 (1960).

36. GREENBERG, J.: Spontaneous arteriovenous malformations in the cervical area. J. Neurol. Neurosurg. Psychiat. 33, 303-309 (197o).

37. HAHN, W.: Gutartige Veränderungen der Mundschleimhaut. Die Quintessenz der zahnärztl. Literatur. Farbbild-Atlas, Bl. 149 Bild 371 (1958).

38. HAMMER, H.: Zur Klinik der Geschwülste im Mund und Kieferbereich besonders in differential und frühdiagnostischer Hinsicht. Deutsche zahnärztl. Zeitschr. 12, 172-191 (1957).

39. HARADA, N., HIRAYAMA, A., SUZUKI, J.: External carotid-intracranial sinus fistulae; a case report and 9 cases of the fistulae in literature. Brain & Nerve (Tokyo) 20, 797-800 (1968).

40. HOUSER, O. W., BAKER, H. L. Jr., RHOTON, A. L., OKAZAKI, H.: Intracranial dural arteriovenous malformations. Radiology 105/1, 55-64 (1972).

41. HUBER, P.: Gefäßmißbildungen und Gefäßtumoren der Arteria Carotis externa und der Dura. Röfo. 109, 325-335 (1968).

42. IRACI, G., CARTERI, A.: Anomalous arterio-venous aneurysm of the middle menigeal artery. Med. Times (N. Y.) 93, 316-320 (1965).

43. KAUFMANN, I.: Objective tinnitus aurium and dural arteriovenous malformations of the posterior fossa. Anals Otol. Rhinol.& Laryngol. 80, 111-122 (1971).

44. KIM, Y. H., GILDENBERG, P. L., DUCHESNEAU, P. M.: Angiographic evidence of spontaneous closure of nontraumatic arteriovenous fistula of the vertebral artery. J. Neurosurg. 38, 658-661 (1973).

45. KRAMER, R., NEWTON, T. H.: Tentorial branches of the internal carotid artery. Am. J. Roentgenol. 95, 826-830 (1965).

46. KRAYENBÜHL, H., YASMARGIL, M. G.: Die vaskulären Erkrankungen im Gebiet der A. vertebralis und A. basilaris: eine anatomische und pathologische, klinische und neuroradiologische Studie, p.145 Stuttgart: Thieme 1957.

47. KRAYENBÜHL, H.: Vaskuläre Krankheiten im extracraniellen Carotis-Vertebralis-Bereich als Ursache intracranieller Geräusche. Münch. Med. Wschr. 103, 2185-2187 (1961).

48. KRAYENBÜHL, H.: The value of orbital angiography for diagnosis of unilateral exophthalmos. J. Neurosurg. 19, 289-301 (1962).

49. KRAYENBÜHL, H., YASARGIL, H. M.: Die zerebrale Angiographie, S. 202. Stuttgart: Thieme 1965.

50. KUNC, Z., BRET, J.: Congenital arterio-sinusal fistulae. Acta Neuro-Chirurg. 20, 85-103 (1969).

51. KURAMOTO, S., WATANABE, M., TAKAMIYA, Y., FUJIKI, H.: A case of traumatic fistula in the superficial temporal artery, anterior cerebral artery and superior sagittal sinus. Brain & Nerve (Tokyo) 19, 91-95 (1967).

52. LAINE, E., GALIBERT, P., LOPEZ, C., DELABROUSSE, J. M., CHRISTIAENS, J. L.: Anéurismes artério-veineux intraduraux de la fossa posteriore. Neuro-Chirurgie 9, 147-158 (1963).

53. LANG, E. K., HETHERINGTON, J. A.: Arteriovenous malformation of the occipital region. J. Indiana Med. Ass. 59, 13-26 (1966).

54. LANGE- COSACK, H.: Anatomie und Klinik der Gefäßmißbildungen des Gehirns und seiner Häute. Handb. d. Neuro-Chirurgie, Vol. 4, Part. 2, 1-45 (1966).

55. LAWSON, Th. L., NEWTON, Th. H.: Congenital cervical arteriovenous malformations. Radiology, 97, 565-570 (1970).

56. LAWTON, R. L., TIDRICK, R. T., BRINTNALL, E. S.: A clinic-pathologic study of multiple congenital arteriovenous fistulae of the lower ectremities. Angiologica 8, 161-172 (1957).

57. LEPOIRE, J., MONTAUT, J., BOUCHOT, M., LAXENAIRE, M.: Anéurysmes artério-veineux intra-frontaux vascularisés par l'artère ethmoidale antérieure. A propos des trois observations. Neuro-Chirurgie 9, 159-166 (1963).

58. LINDEMANN: zit. nach REICHENBACH 1957.

59. MARKHAM, J. W.: Spontaneous arteriovenous fistula of the vertebral artery and vein; case report. J. Neurosurg. 31, 220-223 (1969).

60. MARTIN, J. D., MABON, R. F.: Pulsation exophthalmus: review of all reported cases. M. A. 121, 330 (1943). Zit. nach Verbiest 1968.

61. MATHIS, H.: Gewächse und gewächsartige Bildungen der Mundhöhle und ihrer Umgebung. Die Quintessenz der zahnärztl. Literatur, Farbbild-Atlas, Bl. 36, Bild 74, 75, 76 (1958).

62. MAW, A. R.: Some features of arteriovenous fistula malformations in the head and neck. Laryngoscope 82, 785-795 (1972).

63. MCCORMICK, W. F., BOULTER, T. R.: Vascular malformations ('angiomas') of the dura mater; report of two cases. J. Neurosurg. 25, 309-311 (1966).

64. MCCORMICK, W. F.: The pathology of vascular arteriovenous malformations. J. Neurosurg. 24, 807-816 (1967).

65. METZGER et al.: Zit. nach DEBRUN 1972.

66. MINGRINO, S., MORO, F.: Fistula between the external carotid artery and the cavernous sinus. J. Neurosurg. 27, 157-160, (1967).

67. MONIZ, E., D'ABREU, D., OLIVEIRA, C.: L'aspect à l'épreuve encephalographique des angiomes artériels di cerveau dans le domaine de la carotide interne. Rev. Neurol. 3911, 165 (1932).

68. NEWTON, T. H., DARROCH, J.: Vertebral arteriovenous fistula complicating vertebral angiography. Acta Radiol. (Diag.) 5, 428-440 (1966).

69. NEWTON, T. H., GREITZ, T.: Arteriovenous communication between the occipital artery and transverse sinus. Radiology 87, 842-828 (1966).

70. NEWTON, T. H., WEIDNER, W., GREITZ, T.: Dural arteriovenous malformations in the posterior fossa. Radiology 90, 27-35, (1968).

71. NEWTON, T. H., CHRONQUIST, S.: Involvement of dural arteries in intracaranial arterio-venous malformations. Radiology 93, 1071-1078 (1969).

72. NICOLA, G. C., NIZZOLI, V.: Dural arterio-venous malformations of the posterior fossa. J. Neurol. Neurosurg. Psychiat. 31, 514-519 (1968).

73. NORMAN, J. A., SCHMIDT, K. W., GROW, J. B.: Congenital arteriovenous fistula of the cervical vertebral vessels with heart failure in an infant. J. Pediat. 36, 598-604 (1950).

74. OBRADOR, S., URQUIZA, P.: Angioma artério-veineux de la tente de cervelet. Folia psychiat. neurol. et neurochir. (neerl.) 55, 385-387 (1952).

75. OLIVECRONA, H., LADENHEIM, J.: Congenital arteriovenous aneurysms of the carotid and vertebral arterial systems. 91 pp., 8-9. Berlin: Springer 1957.

76. PECKER, J., BONNAL, J., JAVALET, A.: Deux nouveaux cas d' anévrysmes artério-veineux intraduraux de la fosse postérieure alimentés par la carotide externe. Neuro-Chirurgie 11, 327-332 (1965).

77. PEETERS, F. L., VROOMEN, J. G. H.: Die meningeale Versorgung intracranieller arteriovenöser Mißbildungen. Röfo 113, 303-311 (1971).

78. PERRET, G., NISHIOKA, H.: Report on the cooperative study of intracranial aneurysms and subarachnoid hemorrhage. Section VI. Arteriovenous malformations.An analysis of 545 cases of cranio-cerebral arteriovenous malformations and fistulae reported to the cooperative study. J. Neurosurg. 25, 467-490 (1966).

79. PRADAT, P., DOYON, D., NAVARRO-ARTILLES, G., RAYMOND, J. P.: Anéurysme artério-veineux sous dural de la gouttière olfactive. Neuro-Chirurgie 14, 923-930 (1968).

80. PYGOTT, F., HUTTON, C. F.: Angioma of the neck with intraspinal extension. Brit. J. Radiol. 37, 72-73 (1964).

81. RAMAMURTHI, B., BALASUBRAMANIAN, V.: Arteriovenous malformations with a purely external carotid contribution. Report of two cases. J. Neurosurg. 25, 643-647 (1966).

82. RASKIND, R., WEISS, S. R., DORIA, A.: Nontraumatic fistula cervical portion of vertebral artery and jugular vein. Vase Surg. 1, 224-229 (1967).

83. RAVITCH, M. M., GAERTNER, R. A.: Congenital arteriovenous fistula in the neck - 48 year follow-up of a patient operated upon by Dr. Halsted in 1911. Bull. Johns Hopk. Hosp. 107, 31-56 (1960).

84. REICHENBACH, E.: Verfahren der Blutstillung bei operativen Eingriffen in der Mundhöhle. Deutsche zahnärztl. Zeitschr. 12, 264-276 (1957).

85. REINHOFF, W. F.Jr.: Congenital arteriovenous fistula. An embryological study, with report of a case. Bull. Johns Hopk. Hosp. 35, 271-284 (1924).

86. RICHTER, H. R.: Collaterals between the external carotid artery and the vertebral artery in cases of thrombosis on the internal carotid artery. Acta Radiol. (Diagn.) (Stockh.) 40, 108-112 (1953).

87. ROBINSON, J. L., SEDZIMIR, C. B.:External carotid-transverse sinus fistula. J. Neurosurg. 33, 718-721 (1970).

88. ROBLES, J.: Congenital arteriovenous malformation of the vertebral vessels in the neck. J. Neurosurg. 29, 206-208 (1968).

89. SCHECHTER, M. M., GUTSTEIN, R. A.: Aneurysms and arteriovenous fistulas of the superficial temporal vessels. Radiology 97, 549-557 (1970).

90. SCHUMACKER, H. V. Jr., CAMPBELL, R. L., HEIMBURGER, R. F.: Operative treatment of vertebral arteriovenous fistulas. J. Trauma 6, 3-19 (1966).

91. SENARCLENS, B., SCHAFER, J., WUETHRICH, R.: Von der A. carotis externa ausgehende arteriovenöse Mißbildungen der hinteren Schädelgrube. Schweiz. Arch. Neurol., Neurochir., Psychiat. 110, 69-82 (1972).

92. SHER, M., MEYER, N., LENHARDT, H., TRUMMER, M.: Arteriovenous fistula involving the vertebral artery. Report of three cases. Ann. Surg. 163, 408-413 (1966).

93. SHIGA, H., GAMO, T.: Arteriovenous fistula between the external carotid artery and the transverse sinus. Brain & Nerve 18, 851-853. Tokyo 1965.

94. STATTIN, S.: Meningeal vessels of internal carotid artery and their angiographic significance. Acta Radiol. 55, 513-520 (1963).

95. STORRS, D. G., KING, R. B.: Management of extracranial arteriovenous malformations of the head and neck. J. Neurosurg. 38, 584-590 (1973).

96. SUTTON, D. A., PRATT, E.: Vertebral arterio-venous fistula. Clin. Radiol. 22, 289-295 (1971).

97. SVOLOS, D., NOMIKOS, N., TZOULIADIS, V.: Congenital arteriovenous aneurysms in the neck. J. Neurosurg. 23, 68-71 (1965).

98. TAKAKAWA, S. D., HOLMAN, C. B.: Roentgenologic diagnosis of anomalous communications between external carotid artery and intracranial veins. Am. J. Roentgenol. 95, 822-825 (1965).

99. TAMAKI, N., FUJITA, K., YAMASHITA, H.: Multiple arteriovenous malformations involving the scalp, dura, retina, cerebrum and posterior fossa. Case report. J. Neurosurg., 34, 95-98 (1971).

100. TERAO, H., HAYAKAWA, I.: Arteriovenous fistula between the external carotid artery and the sigmoid sinus; case report. Clinical Neurology (Tokyo) 3, 122-126 (1963).

101. TÖNNIS, W.: In: Bergstrand, H., OLIVECRONA, H., Tönnis, W.: Gefäßmißbildungen und Gefäßgeschwülste des Gehirns. 88-134-181. Leipzig: Thieme 1936.

102. TSUJI, H. K.: Unpublished-mentioned in J. thor. cardiovasc. Surg. 55, 746-753 (1968).

103. VAN BUREN, J., POPPE, L., HOVRAX, G.: Unilateral Exophthalmus. A consideration of symptom pathogenesis. Brain 80, 139-175 (1957).

104. VAN DER WERF, A. J.: Sur un cas d'anévrisme artério-veineux interdural bilatéral de la fosse posterieure chez un enfant. Neuro-Chirurgie (Paris) 10, 140-144 (1964).

105. VAN WIJNGAARDEN, G. K., VINKEN, P. J.: Case of intradural arteriovenous aneurysm of the posterior fossa. Neurology 16, 754-756 (1966).

106. VERBIEST, M. H.: L'anévrisme artérioveineux intradural. Rev. Neurol. 85, 189-199 (1951).

107. VERBIEST, H.: Arterial and arteriovenous aneurysms of the posterior fossa. Psychiat. Neurol. Neurochir. 65, 329-369 (1962).

108. VERBIEST, H.: Extracranial and cervical arteriovenous aneurysms of the carotid and vertebral arteries. Report of a series of 12 personal cases. Johns Hopk. Med. J. 122, 350-357 (1968).

109. WEIDAUER, H.: Ein Beitrag zu objektiv wahrnehmbaren Ohrgeräuschen. Zschr. Laryngol. Rhinol. Otol. 49, 227-230 (1970).

110. YASARGIL, M. G.: Die Röntgendiagnostik des Exophthalmus unilateralis, 1 Vol. Basel: Karger 1957.

111. ZIKLHA, A., SCHECHTER, M. M.: Arteriovenous fistulas of the major of the neck. Acta Radiol. (Diagn.) 9, 560-572 (1969).

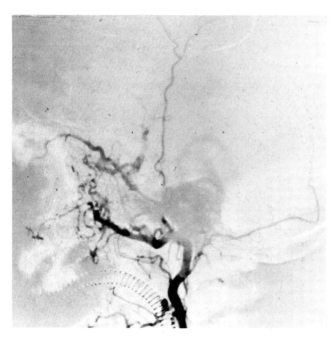

Fig. 1. P. C., 3 years old, F. Selective external carotid angiography.
Arteriovenous angioma of the left side of the face, supplied by branches from the external carotid artery. Main feeder: Internal maxillary
artery

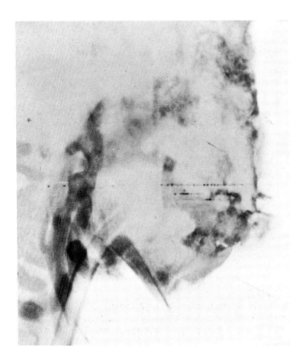

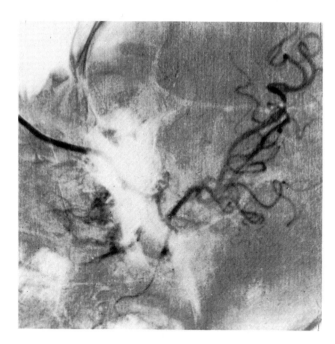

Fig. 3. Same patient. Selective angiography of the internal carotid artery. Filling of the Sylvian artery territory only

◀Fig. 2. M. A., 12 years, M. Common carotid angiography. Dilatation of the common carotid and external carotid arteries. Arteriovenous angioma of the left side of the face. Supply from all branches of the external carotid artery

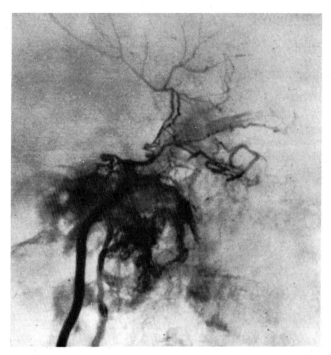

Fig. 4. Same patient. Angiography performed after both the external carotid arteries had been ligated. Angioma supplied by the branches of the ophthalmic artery. No filling of intracranial vessels on the left side. Steal syndrome

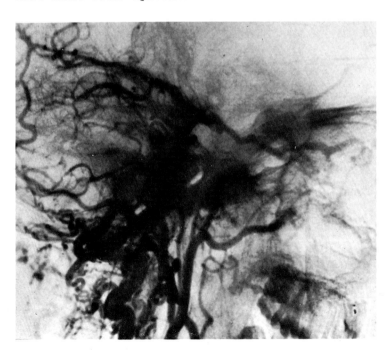

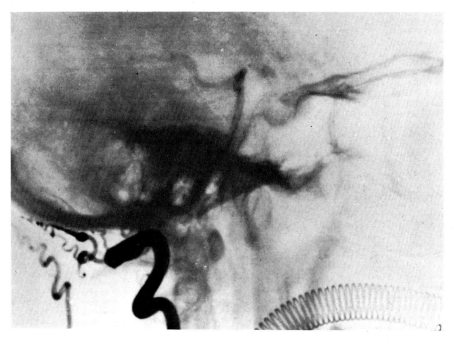

Fig. 6. Ü. L., 56 years, F. Left sided brachial angiography. Arterio-venous angioma of the cervico-occipital region. Intracranial extension supplied by the meningeal branches of the vertebral artery

◄Fig. 5. Same patient. Right vertebral angiography. Angioma supplied by the occipital artery and branches of the vertebral artery. Dilated posterior communicating artery, which continues directly into the ophthalmic artery

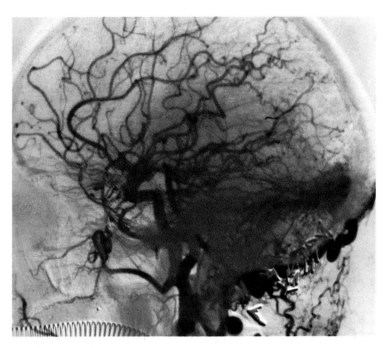

Fig. 7. Same patient. Incomplete microsurgical extirpation of the angioma on the left side. Right brachial angiography. Angioma supplied by the thyro-cervical trunk, right vertebral and occipital artery with intracranial extension of the malformation

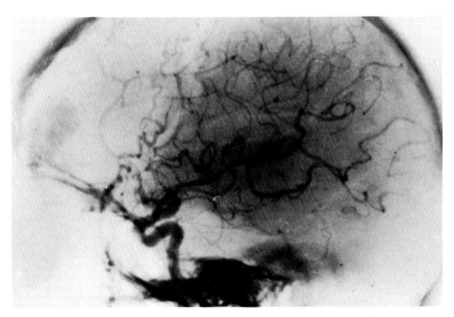

Fig. 8. S. B., 4o years, F. Arteriovenous angioma supplied by the ethmoidal artery, drainage into the intracranial paramedial frontal vein

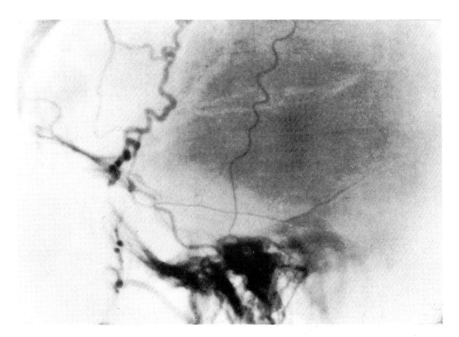

Fig. 9. Same patient. Selective external carotid artery angiography.
Malformation supplied through the meningeal branches of the external
carotid artery. Drainage through intracranial paramedian frontal vein

Discussion on Chapter III

HEKSTER: I would like to congratulate Dr. DJINDJIAN once again on his extremely beautiful and extraordinarily good embolizations. Recently there have been several reports by plastic surgeons on the treatment of angiomas of the face with large doses of corticosteroids. The results, so far as can be judged by photographs, are extraordinarily good. We have had the opportunity of treating a small child with decompensation of the heart due to shunting, who had such an angioma, with large doses of Cortisone, and we are quite happy with the result.

WALDER: (to DJINDJIAN) Is it possible to have small catheters with a small balloon at the tip, which one can introduce into the intracerebral arteries?

DJINDJIAN: I hope we will be able to do this one day. So far it is still impossible for me.

BECK: (to DJINDJIAN) What complications have you encountered with your method?

DJINDJIAN: Embolization is a very easy technique, and that it is why it is necessary to be very careful. The complications are local ones, especially in the region of the tragus, and of the nose, and in the tongue. With large emboli you may get necrosis. Surgeons experience the same complications, when ligating the vessels.

Another complication can occur, if too many emboli are used. In such cases the last emboli may return with the back-flow into the internal carotid. This is why we use only small strips of gelfoam, because it is the thrombus which forms around gelfoam which is responsible for good embolization.

As far as the magnification technique is concerned, I found it to be an extremely useful adjunct to superselective angiography, enabling one to see vessels of 100 to 200 microns in diameter.

Chapter IV
Pathophysiological Aspects

The Influence of Cerebral Steal: Demonstration by Fluorescein
Angiography and Focal Cerebral Blood Flow Measurement

W. FEINDEL

The   Recognition   of   Cerebral   Steal   as
a   Factor   in   Cerebral   Angiomas

Despite the reports of many excellent results from the surgery of cerebral angiomas, summarized by many writers including POOL and POTTS
(1), FRENCH and CHOU (2), our basic understanding of the hemodynamic
mechanisms and the dramatic disturbances in the cerebral circulation
associated with angiomas is still very imprecise.

Some of the main principles in the surgical approach to these lesions
were established in the earliest reports of CUSHING and BAILEY (3),
DANDY (4), and BERGSTRAND, OLIVECRONA and TÖNNIS (5). They reported
the following points:

1. Arteriovenous shunting of red arterial blood into the draining veins
   was seen at operation.

2. The unsatisfactory therapeutic effect of ligating extracranial arterial vessels.

3. The uncertain therapeutic results of ligating some but not all of
   the cerebral arterial feeding vessels.

4. The importance of interrupting the arterial feeders and avoiding
   the draining veins during the surgical removal of the angioma.

While hemorrhage from arteriovenous malformations has been recognized
as a surgical emergency, calling often for heroic measures, it has also been appreciated over many years that the relentless neurological
deficit and mental deterioration as well as epileptic seizures are associated with arteriovenous malformations. The basis of this has not
been clear in any detailed way. Nor do we understand why occasionally
these potentially devastating lesions have a surprisingly benign course
over a period of many years.

Elsewhere, we have reviewed in detail the historical background and
our own evidence for the "cerebral steal syndrome" (6). It had long
been demonstrated by angiography that cerebral angiomas were related
to a rapid circulation time with early filling of cerebral veins and
relatively poor filling of the normal arterial branches, as described,

* The development of the technique reported here was supported by grants
  from the medical research council of Canada and the cone memorial fund
  of the Montreal neurological institute.

for example, by ELVIDGE (7) in 1938. A number of other early studies, particularly those by NORLÉN (8) and BESSMAN and his associates (9), indicated further that there was better filling of the normal cerebral arteries following obliteration or excision of the angioma. These observations were confirmed by many other surgeons and radiologists over the years as angiographic techniques became more refined. Nevertheless, this was a relatively crude indication of the degree of circulatory shunting and of the effect it might have on the surrounding brain, since the findings were limited to arterial vessels proximal to the microcirculation. However, this shunt flow was interpreted by many as an indication of some type of impairment of the circulation of the surrounding normal brain, and it was MURPHY (10) in 1954 who seems to have been the first to use the term "steal" in this connection.

With the introduction of radio-active isotopic techniques for studying the cerebral circulation, it was possible to establish a quantitative approach to this problem. Using scintillation detectors on the neck and at various sites over the head, we were able to show that the peak of radio-activity after intravenous injection of a non-diffusible isotope appeared almost simultaneously at the head and the neck, with the carotid-jugular time being shortened from a normal of 8 seconds to 2 seconds and the flow peaks giving a higher rate over the angioma as compared to normal areas of brain (11). At the same time it was noted that the radio-isotopic brain scan indicated an early positive uptake over an angioma as compared to the later uptake of tumors or infarcts (12, 21). These early findings were confirmed by many other workers, including MAYNARD and associates (13) and ROSENTHAL (14).

Further evidence for the physiological disturbance associated with the shunting flow of the cerebral angioma was obtained by PEROT and myself in 1965 from direct observations of the angioma during operation and by measuring transit time curves with radio-isotopic tracers from the surface of the brain (15). We modified Murphy's term to "cerebral steal", as being appropriate to the description of the rapid shunt flow through an angioma going directly from the arterial to the venous system and related to a reduction in circulation to the surrounding normal cortex. We classified the various situations in which red cerebral veins were noted to appear (but the variety of other lesions associated with red veins need not concern us here). In general, in addition to the direct arteriovenous connections, they indicate in most instances a loss of autoregulation, either locally or generally, of the normal control of cerebral blood flow. Thus, for the first time the evidence for cerebral steal could be put on a quantitative basis and the changes from shunt flow to perfusion flow could be measured during surgery (16). Closure of the main arterial input to the angioma was, of course, followed by a reduction in the amplitude and the prolongation of the radio-isotope flow curve. Later findings by OECONOMOS and others (17) using extracranial monitoring with radio-isotopes confirmed our observations. An important characteristic which we noted was the loss of the "shunt peak" of the transit time curves and the clearance curves of the radio-isotopic tracers, as monitored from the surface of the brain before and after reduction or cessation of the shunt flow. At the same time, we noted an increase of the perfusion flow in the surrounding normal brain, as measured directly from the surface of the brain during operation (18).

F l u r o e s c e i n   A n g i o g r a p h i c   F i n d i n g s

Visual evidence for the conversion of the cerebral steal shunt flow into improved perfusion flow was provided when we introduced the use of fluorescein angiography of the brain for the investigation of these complex lesions during operation. The early filling of the shunting veins by the fluorescent dye could be noted on rapid serial color photography, ciné film or television. The red veins were seen to fill much earlier than the normal veins and to present a mixing or swirling flow in contrast to the well-defined laminar streaking flow in the veins draining the normal regions of the cortex. In addition, fluorescein angiography made it possible for the first time to examine the microcirculation directly. The cerebral steal was demonstrated by the change in distribution and intensity of the fluorescein dye in the cortical microcirculation before and after reduction or obliteration of the arteriovenous shunt through the angioma. This increase in microregional blood flow was seen to correspond to the changes identified quantitatively by the radio-active Xenon clearance studies and the non-diffusible isotopic transit time measurements.

F e a t u r e s   o f   t h e   C e r e b r a l   S t e a l   S y n - d r o m e

In a previous report (6, 18) we summarized the most notable features of the cerebral steal syndrome. These were based on our early studies with radio-isotopic measurements both extracranial and during operation directly from the cortex, from the study of vascular flow patterns on the surface of the brain using either Coomassie Blue dye (16) or fluorescein angiography (19, 20). These observations have made it possible to substantiate the earlier suggestion of the "steal" related solely to arteriographic findings which were largely non-quantitative and gave no evidence relating directly to the microcirculation or perfusion flow. The main features of the syndrome are:

1. Rapid brain circulation transit time and short carotid-jugular interval as measured by radio-isotopes.

2. Early positive uptake on the radio-active brain scan.

3. Hyperoxemia of the jugular venous blood.

4. Early filling of veins and relatively poor filling of normal arteries as well as cross-over flow from the opposite side on angiography.

5. At craniotomy filling of red veins with mixing and pulsating arterial blood under increased pressure and increased oxygen levels. Occlusion of the arterial supply or excision of the malformation causes these red veins to turn blue and to exhibit more normal laminar flow.

6. High non-nutritional non-perfusion shunt flow through the malformation into the draining veins.

7. Conversion of shunt flow to perfusion flow after obliteration of the vessels supplying the angioma or after excision of the angioma. The shunt peaks on the isotopic curves disappear, perfusion flow in the surrounding brain improves, and the transit time curves are prolonged. In addition, fluorescein angiography demonstrates improved flow through the microcirculation of the adjacent brain.

8. These circulatory findings support the view that progressive symptoms and signs associated with arteriovenous malformations, such as focal seizures, memory impairment, sensory and motor deficit, and mental deterioration, are the clinical correlates of a cerebral steal syndrome which can occur without hemorrhage or thrombosis.

9. The firm evidence now established for the role of the cerebral steal syndrome in angiomas makes this a strong indication for surgical

treatment of these complex lesions, quite aside from the presence
of hemorrhage or evidence of vascular occlusion. In some patients
increased intracranial pressure resulting from the transfer of arterial pressure to the venous system with headaches and papilloede-
ma serves as a further feature of the malformation which demands
surgical treatment.

A   Note   on   Techniques

The measurement of microregional cerebral blood flow directly from the
brain originated from the rather crude extracranial methods which we
first used in 1956 (11, 12) by designing new miniature gamma-sensitive
detectors from lithium-drifted silicon (20). These measure the gamma
activity mainly from the width of a single convolution and allow for
transit time as well as clearance studies (Figs. 1, 2). Registration
of the gamma activity is put through a PDP-12 computer with a display
terminal in the operating room providing on-line values for the multiple cortical areas being examined during operation. Identification
of the shunt peak in and around the angioma and obliteration of this
peak with improvement of the perfusion flow can be observed by the
surgeon during operation as an index of the degree of obliteration of
the "cerebral steal".

The use of fluorescein angiography in the operating room has given
visual display of these quantitative changes. Using direct or overhead
photography through a mirror (19, 20), the system provides for permanent photographic color pictures of the blood flow patterns in the
epicerebral circulation or for television which can be replayed for the
surgeon during operation, and during which polaroid black-and-white
pictures can be taken for direct comparison with different phases of
the circulation of the exposed operative field. As we have noted before (16, 20), the identification of the multiple feeding arteries
from amongst the complex leash of arteries and red veins makes it possible for the surgeon to carry out precise selective arterial oblider-
ation of the angioma with the preservation of the blood supply to the
normal surrounding brain. This allows us to deal with complex angiomas
adjacent to the sensory motor or speech areas which otherwise would be
considered inoperable.

In making the flow studies, the radio-active tracers and the fluorescein dye are injected by way of a catheter selectively placed in the
internal carotid artery (Fig. 3).

C a s e   R e p o r t

Case 1. H. L. (30 years of age). This patient had acute hemorrhage from
an arteriovenous malformation in the left parietal region. After recovery from coma and dysphasia, craniotomy and excision of the malformation were carried out (March, 1963). Transit time curves with Hip-
puran Iodine[125] before and after clipping of some of the major supply
to the angioma by way of two large branches from the anterior cerebral
artery demonstrated a prolongation and reduction of the large shunt
curve measured from the angioma.

Case 2. R. G. (30 years of age). This patient complained of numbness
for a period of about ten hours in the left hand and left face ten days

before admission to hospital (January,1968). Three days after the on-set, he had a focal seizure involving the left side of the body. An-giography showed a small pea-sized angioma in the lower central region on the right side with an early filling central vein. At operation, the central vein was red. There was no evidence on the surface of the pres-ence of an angioma or of any ischemic area, although electrocortico-graphy from the post-central gyrus, identified by electrical stimula-tion, showed slow waves. It was only during cerebral fluorescein an-giography that a distinct impairment of microcirculatory flow could be shown in this post-central region. Two examples taken from the rap-id serial fluorescein angiographic photographs demonstrate this. At 1.99 seconds the central vein is already filling with fluorescein while the remaining epicerebral veins are seen to be dark and unfilled with dye (Fig. 4). The post-central convolution fills very slowly and a re-gion of cortex on either side of the central vein as it ascends toward the longitudinal sinus also shows poor filling with the dye. Thus, we have the combination of the shunt flow in the central vein, in which the swirling flow was displayed by the fluorescein, associated with the region of poor filling of the cortical microcirculation.

At 5.26 seconds the reverse of the earlier fluorescein picture is present, that is, the fluorescein dye has not yet cleared from the post-central convolution while the microcirculation in the rest of the hemisphere shows almost complete washout of the dye (Fig. 5). In addi-tion, one notes again the filling of the red central vein with fluor-escein, with little evidence of laminar flow. In the other veins, the laminar flow derived from the terminal branches of the veins joining the larger collecting veins is quite distinct. The most significant feature is the density of the fluorescein in the microcirculation of the post-central gyrus. It was possible on sequential photographs taken at intervals of 3/10 of a second and from ciné film to determine that the flow into this post-central cortex was by way of back flow coming downward in the epicerebral arteries from the anterior cerebral dis-tribution. This area of focal ischemia demonstrated so clearly by flu-orescein angiography was measured also by Xenon clearance studies and by non-diffusible radio-isotope transit time curves. The post-central cortex showed the lowest flow values. A shunt peak was identified over the region of the small angioma on the isotope studies, with a smaller peak recorded over the red central vein.

These findings could be interpreted in the following way. The angioma and a small subcortical hematoma had produced the sudden onset of is-chemia in the sensory area related to the arm and face. This focal is-chemia could be partly due to the shunt flow with the cerebral steal and partly due to the compression of the overlying cortex by the hema-toma. It was noted that following removal of the hematoma the slow waves were reduced in amplitude and in the area of distribution. The removal of the hematoma was, of course, made at the same time that the small angioma was clipped and removed. The potential for recovery of such an ischemic area of cortex was demonstrated by the fact that in the next six years the patient remained free of seizures and had nor-mal discriminatory sensation in his left hand. The association of the cerebral steal and the focal cortical ischemia with focal epileptic seizures is thus well documented.

Case 3. F. K. (age 20 years). She had a large left frontal angioma which had been associated in the preceding two and one-half years with generalized seizures. The arterial supply was complex, coming from the deep and epicerebral branches of the middle and anterior cerebral ar-teries (Fig. 6 a). It was situated just in front of the motor cortex and just superior to the speech cortex. Pre-operative radio-isotopic studies showed a focal uptake in the region of the angioma, while gamma camera studies showed a rapid and high shunt peak over the angioma as compared to the normal hemisphere. A characteristic early positive uptake on the brain scan, as we had noted in earlier reports (12), was also found (21).

At operation fluorescein angiography made it possible to identify the feeding arteries to this complex lesion (Figs. 6 b, 6 c). For example, it was possible to define an artery crossing the motor cortex and to occlude the distal portion of this vessel while preserving the supply to the important cortical region. In this instance, the fluorescein angiography was played back to the surgeon on video-tape and provided also by polaroid pictures so that each stage of the selective obliteration of the arteries could be followed.

The fluorescein studies also gave a dramatic indication of the reversal of the shunt flow to perfusion flow into the surrounding normal brain. For example, at 1 second following partial obliteration of the arterial input the microcirculation of the inferior frontal, temporal and parietal cortex was much more evident. This became even more notable at a slightly later phase of the angiogram at 1.8 seconds (Table 1 a, b). Xenon clearance studies confirmed quantitatively this visual picture so that the microregional flow through the speech cortex which was 0.641 units before occlusion of the feeding arteries became 0,926 units or an increase of 44% after the obliteration of the arteries. The shunt peak which had been recorded from the parietal and frontal cortex were obliterated. Post-operative angiography showed marked reduction in the extent of the angiomatous lesion. She had no post-operative neurological deficit and no seizures in the 3 years since operation.

Summary

1. The features of the cerebral steal syndrome have been described.
2. Using radio-isotopic measurement of cerebral blood flow extracranially and during operation, together with fluorescein angiography of the epicerebral circulation, we have been able to show reduction in the shunt flow and improvement of the perfusion flow through the microcirculation of the cerebral cortex following obliteration or excision of the arteriovenous malformations.
3. These combined techniques thus provide a firm basis for the cerebral steal syndrome and at the same time enable the surgeon to carry out a more precise excision of the angioma using flow values and angiography on television as a guide during operation.
4. Our original concept of the cerebral steal syndrome has thus been substantiated by more recent findings. The presence of cerebral steal is a strong indication for operative treatment of cerebral angiomas even in the absence of clinical evidence of hemorrhage or thrombosis, in order to prevent the relentless progression of neurological deficit, mental deterioration and epileptic seizures.

Acknowledgement

The author wishes to thank Dr. Lucas Yamamoto and Mr. Charles Hodge for their collaboration in this work which has been reviewed in certain aspects elsewhere, and to Mr. George Lootus and Mrs. Andrea Duzycyzyn for expert technical help.

Table 1 a and b. a) Change in the shunt peak noted on the transit time curves in patient F. K. before and after arterial occlusion. b) Increase in blood flow calculated as perfusion flow before and after occlusion of the feeding arteries to the angioma

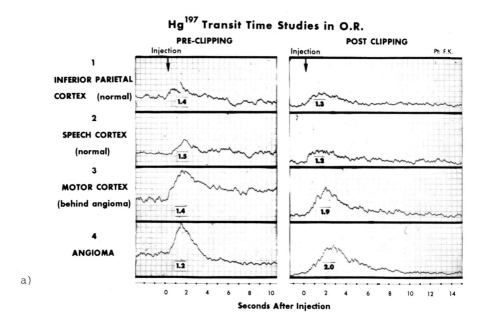

a)

Xenon Clearance Studies in O.R.

F.K.

Probe Location	Blood Flow Rate F/λ (infinity value)	
	Before clipping of feeding arteries to angioma	After clipping of feeding arteries to angioma
Inferior Parietal Cortex (normal)	0.932	0.996 (+7%)
Speech Cortex (normal)	0.641	0.926 (+44%)
Motor Cortex (behind angioma)	0.682	1.040 (+52%)
Angioma Area	0.349	1.190 (+241%)
pCO₂	41	42
B.P.	110	80

b)

References

1. POOL, J. L., POTTS, D. G.: Aneurysms and Arteriovenous Anomalies of the Brain: Diagnosis and Treatment. New York: Harper & Row 1965.

2. FRENCH, L. A., CHOU, S. N.: Conventional methods of treating intracranial arteriovenous malformations. Prog. Neurol. Surg. 3, 274-319 (1969).

3. CUSHING, H., BAILEY, P.: Tumours Arising from the Blood Vessels of the Brain: Angiomatous Malformations and Haemangioblastomas. Springfield, Ill.:Charles C. Thomas 1928.

4. DANDY, W. E.: Venous abnormalities and angiomas of the brain. Arch. Surg. 17, 715-793, 1928.

5. BERGSTRAND, H., OLIVECRONA, H., TÖNNIS, W.: Gefässmissbildungen und Gefässgeschwulste des Gehirns. Leipzig: Georg Thieme 1936.

6. FEINDEL, W., YAMAMOTO, Y. L., HODGE, C. P.: Red Cerebral Veins and the Cerebral Steal Syndrome: Evidence from fluorescein angiography and microregional blood flow by radioisotopes during excision of an angioma. J. Neurosurg. 35, 167-179 (1971).

7. ELVIDGE, A. R.: The cerebral vessels studied by angiography. In: Penfield, W. (ed.): The Circulation of the Brain and Spinal Cord, p. 110-149. Baltimore: Williams and Wilkins Co. 1938.

8. NORLEN, G.: Arteriovenous aneurysms of the brain: a report of ten cases of total removal of the lesion. J. Neurosurg. 6, 475-494 (1949).

9. BESSMAN, A. N., HAYES, G. J., ALMAN, R. W., et al.:Cerebral hemodynamics in cerebral arteriovenous vascular anomalies: report of two cases. Med. Ann. D. C. 21, 422-466 (1952).

10. MURPHY, J. P.: Cerebrovascular Disease. Chicago: Year Book Publishers 1954.

11. FEDORUK, S., FEINDEL, W.: Measurement of brain circulation time of radio-active iodinated albumin. Can. J. Surg. 3, 312-318 (1960).

12. FEINDEL, W.: Detection of intracranial lesions by contour brain scanning with radioisotopes. Postgrad Med. 31, 15-22 (1962).

13. MAYNARD, C. O., WITCOFSKY, R. L., JANEWAY, R.: Radioisotope arteriography as an adjunct to the brain scan. Radiol. 92, 908-812 (1969).

14. ROSENTHAL, L.:Detection of altered cerebral arterial blood flow using Technitium-99 m Pertechnetate and the gamma ray scintillation camera. Radiol. 88, 713-718 (1967).

15. FEINDEL, W., PEROT, P.: Red cerebral veins: a report on arteriovenous shunts in tumors and cerebral scars. J. Neurosurg. 22, 315. 325 (1965).

16. GARRETSON, H., PEROT, P., YAMAMOTO, Y. L. et al.: Intracarotid Coomassie blue dye as an aid in the surgery of intracranial vascular lesions. J. Neurosurg 26, 577-583 (1967).

17. OECONOMOS, D., KOSMAOGLU, B., PROSSALENTIS, A.: CFB studies in patients with arteriovenous malformations of the brain. In: Brock, M., Fieschi, C., Ingvar, D. H., et al. (eds.): Cerebral Blood Flow: Clinical and Experimental Results. p. 146-148. New York: Springer-Verlag 1969.

18. FEINDEL, W., YAMAMOTO, Y. L., HODGE, C. P.: Red cerebral veins as an index of cerebral steal. Scand. J. Lab. Clin. Invest. 22, Suppl. 102, X: C (1968).

19. FEINDEL, W., YAMAMOTO, Y. L., HODGE, C. P.: Intracarotid fluorescein angiography: A new method for examination of the epicerebral circulation in man. Can. Med. Ass. J. 96, 1-7 (1967).

20. FEINDEL, W., YAMAMOTO, Y. L., HODGE, C. P.: The Cerebral Microcirculation in Man: Analysis by radioisotopic microregional flow measurement and fluorescein angiography. Clin. Neurosurg. 18, 225-245 (1971).

21. YAMAMOTO, Y. L., FEINDEL, W.: Contour brain scanning and radioisotopic circulation studies for differentiating cerebrovascular lesions and tumors. In: Bakay, L. and Klein, D. M. (eds.): Brain Tumor Scanning with Radioisotopes, p. 141-167. Springfield, Ill.: Charles C. Thomas 1969.

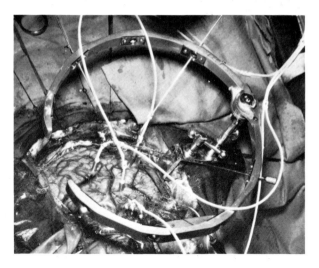

Fig. 1. Array of four miniature solid state gamma-sensitive detectors placed on the cortex at operation. These register radio-isotopic levels after injection of the tracer into the internal carotid artery by means of a catheter

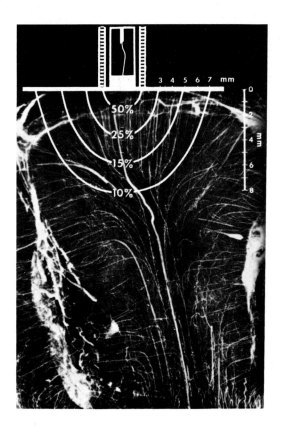

Fig. 2. Outline of the miniature detector shown in relation to a micro-angiogram of a human cerebral convolution. The iso-contour lines indicate the percentage of count rate which the detector registers from the tissue just beneath it

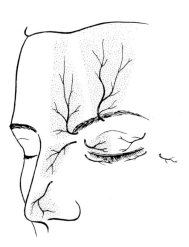

Fig. 3. Drawing to show the cutaneous branches of the ophthalmic artery where a dye blush can be seen when the injection is made by a catheter placed correctly in the internal carotid artery

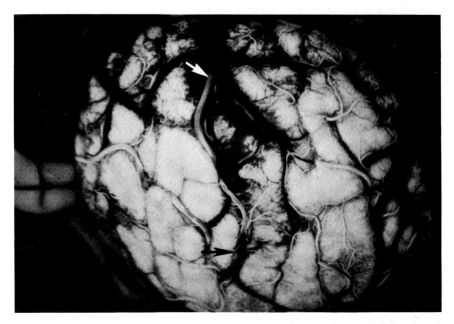

Fig. 4. Fluorescein angiography in patient R. G. At 1.99 secs. after injection the dark central area represents ischemia in the sensory cortex to the left of which, the central vein displays early filling with the fluorescein dye. Note the dark appearance of the normal veins. The white arrow points to the central vein. The black arrow indicates the site of the small angioma

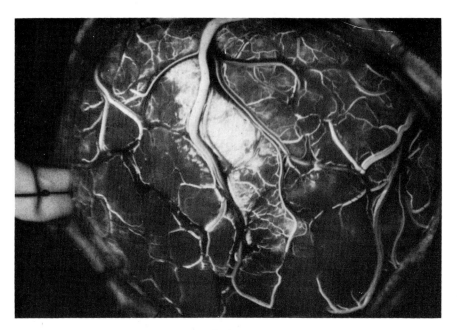

Fig. 5. In the same patient R. G., a photograph of the fluorescein angiogram at 5.2 secs. from the onset shows clearance of the dye from most of the cortex but slow clearing from the sensory cortex. Note the dense dye in the central vein and laminar flow in the nearby normal veins

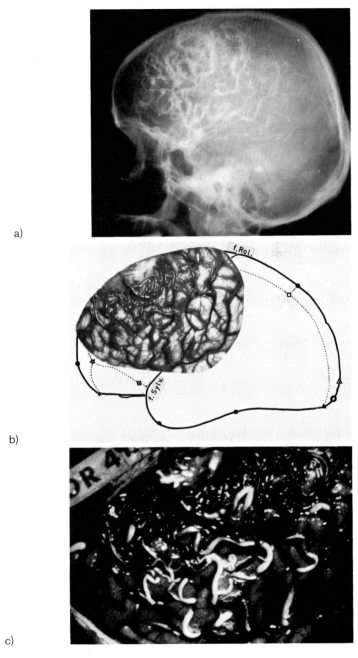

a)

b)

c)

Fig. 6. a) Arterial phase showing the angioma in patient F. K.
b) Montage showing the angioma exposed at operation. c) Early phase
of the fluorescein angiogram showing the individual feeding arteries.
This is a polaroid picture taken from the video playback of the television recording of the fluorescein angiogram

Investigation on Volume and Pressure Overloading of the Heart in Cerebral Angiomas

B. L. Bauer, B. Beck and U. Mössler

Introduction

The neurosurgeon and the cardiologist are both interested in the question to what extent the presence of an arteriovenous malformation is reflected in the function of the heart subject to chronic overloading, and whether it can lead to cardiac failure.

We were stimulated by what is known about cardiac disturbances resulting from the presence of arteriovenous fistulae: increase of the cardiac output, increase of blood volume, and reduction of the circulation time. Moreover, shunt values depend upon the pressure gradient between artery and vein, and from the size and location of the fistula. The increase of cardiac output and consequently that of the cardiac index, is characterized by increased stroee volumes associated with increased heart rate. In experimental arteriovenous fistulae coronary circulation and myocardial uptake of oxygen are increased whereas the coronary vascular resistance is diminished. The blood volume is usually increased, especially when cardiac insufficiency has already developed. It has been proved experimentally that the increase of blood volume is connected with an increase of the plasma fraction. Circulation time is reduced due to the presence of the short-circuit. The combination of increased speed of circulation and increased blood volume is responsible for the increased venous return. The result, as stated above, is an increased cardiac output.

As long as there is no cardiac insufficiency, the venous pressure remains normal. We do not possess any long-term observations on the influence of cerebral arteriovenous malformations upon cardiac function, especially upon the volume and pressure overloading of the heart. So we will have to consider as an analogy the physiological and pathophysiological results observed in cases with persistent ductus-arteriosus (BOTALLI) which may be regarded as a typical congenital arteriovenous fistula. Furthermore, certain data can be obtained from studies in experimentally produced peripheral - not cerebral - arteriovenous fistulae.

According to BING (1), the average shunt volume in cases of persistent ductus arteriosus amounts to 40% of the blood volume pumped through the left ventricle. According to other authors, KEYS et al. (2) and EPPINGER and collaborators (3), these values can reach even 60 to 70%.

Such data indicate the high volume of the overloading of the heart. They also explain the infrequent occurrence of cardiac failure in neonates and children with this defect. We shall discuss this aspect later while speaking about cerebral arteriovenous angiomas. However, one should not forget that the life-expectancy in patients with that anomaly and the same shunt volume, in whom no secondary complications such as endocarditis occur, may be absolutely normal.

LOOGEN (5) was able to demonstrate that the volume overloading need not necessarily produce, as was previously supposed, an increase of the pulmonary flow resistance and a pressure increase in the pulmonary circulation with overloading of the right heart (Table 1).

Table 1. Relation between flow resistance and perfusion rate in the pulmonary circulation in 50 cases of ductus arteriosus apertus (5). (F. LOOGEN, 1958)

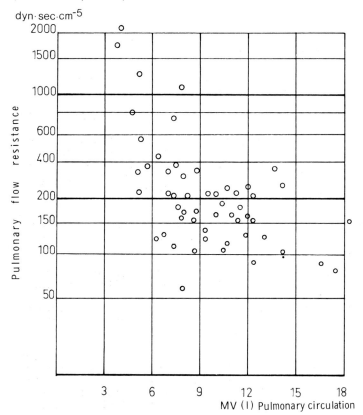

The diagram shows the relation between the pulmonary flow resistance and the volume of the pulmonary circulation in patients with persistent ductus arteriosus. It appears, even, that the pulmonary flow volume is associated with diminished flow resistance. Similar results can be obtained in healthy subjects with a normal pulmonary vascular bed during ergometric stress. If these hemodynamic data are considered in relation to adult patients harbouring a cerebral arteriovenous malformation, it cannot be expected that the critical value of 101 per min. per m^2 of body surface will be seen even in cases with an increased shunt volume and aggravated overloading of the right heart.

The end-diastolic increase of pressure in the right ventricle with corresponding increase in the right atrium could only be expected in cases with an already existing myocardial insufficiency and chronic volume overloading.

The above mentioned pathophysiological findings associated with pressure and volume overloading of the heart and seen in patients with arteriovenous fistulas are characterized mainly by the signs of cardiac insufficiency. One would expect to find them in congenital and acquired cerebral arteriovenous angiomas. We will not discuss here the well-known machinery murmur with slight accentuation of the systolic phase and coexistent thrill, which is so frequently noticed by the patients themselves. The clinical picture is characterized by increase of the cardiac size due to the volume overloading and finally by cardiac insufficiency.

Notes on Techniques and Results

7 patients with cerebral angiomas were the subject of the study. Pressures, oxygen saturation, and circulation time were measured.

Pressures were measured preoperatively through catheterization of the right heart from the right and left basilic veins. The pressure in the large thoracic vessels, right atrium, right ventricle, and the pulmonary artery and pulmonary capillaries (PC-pressure) were estimated. Bloodsamples for estimation of oxygen saturation were drawn from the aorta (Sellinger-catheter), pulmonary artery, right ventricle, right atrium, superior and inferior vena cava, and from subclavian and jugular veins bilaterally (Fig. 1).

Recirculation time was estimated with a precise ascorbic acid dilution method. Ascorbic acid was injected through a catheter into the right ventricle, and its appearance in the jugular veins was measured (Fig. 2).

A catheter electrode was used and the oxidation of reduced indicator - in our case ascorbic acid - was measured proximal and distal to the shunt. The diagrams show the position of the catheter in the right ventricle; in the lower part we see the curve of the ascorbic acid dilution with a recirculation wave 12.1 sec. after the beginning of the injection. This figure represents normal conditions.

In the majority of patients a high oxygen saturation of the blood samples taken from the jugular veins was found. There was no significant difference between the sides and no correlation with the side of the angioma. Relatively high values of oxygen saturation were also found in the inferior cava vein. In no case was the arterial blood undersaturated (Table 2).

Cardiac output - estimated according to the FICK's method - was at the upper limits of normal in three cases and was slightly increased in a further 2 patients. These findings were reflected in the arteriovenous O_2-difference. The recirculation time was considerably reduced in 3 cases, and the mean pulmonary arterial pressure - shown in the diagram on the right side - was slightly increased in 3 cases (Table 3).

This figure shows the recirculation time in 2 patients with angiomas of different size. The upper curve shows the recirculation time in a healthy subject. In the case depicted in the middle of the table there

Table 2. O_2-saturation of blood sampled from big thoracic vessels in patients with cerebral angiomas

I-Number	Subcl. Vein	Jug. Vein	VCS	VCI	PA	Aorta
200445602	82.5	88.5	86.0	85.0	84.5	98.5
020447681	78.0	86.0	82.0	79.5	80.5	96.5
131134631	79.5	84.0	81.0	82.0	82.5	96.5
040140591	75.5	77.0	75.0	80.0	77.0	94.5
220813161	69.5	81.5	75.5	72.0	76.0	96.0
050826131	71.5	78.1	76.5	75.5	75.5	98.0
280561442	84.5	88.5	84.5	83.5	82.5	98.5

Table 3. Circulation values and pressures in patients with cerebral angiomas

I-Number	Cardiac output l/min	Cardiac Index l/min/m²	Arterio-Venous O_2-Difference	Recirculation time of Ascorbic Acid sec	PA/p_m/mm Hg
200445602	7.0[+]	4.1	3.2	7.1[++]	20[+]
020447681	8.9[++]	4.7	3.9	8.0[++]	22[++]
131134631	7.8[++]	4.3	3.5	9[++]	17
040140591	4.8	2.7	3.7	11	13
220813161	7.0[+]	3.6	4.6	12	19[+]
280561442	6.6[+]	4.9	2.7	-	15
050826131	4.9	2.6	5.2	-	14

+   Upper limit of normal.
++ Increased/recirculation time reduced.
PA Pulmonary artery.

was a moderate sized angioma, and the recirculation time of 9.2 sec. was evidently reduced. Further reduction of the recirculation time down to 7.1 sec. was revealed in a patient with a huge cerebral angioma, depicted in the lower part of the table. There seems to exist a certain dependence of recirculation time upon the size of the angioma. However, the number of cases examined is insufficient (Fig. 3).

Case Report

A 2 years and 2 months old boy was first seen in autumn 1970. During the general examination a heart murmur was found, and the boy was referred to us with the suspicion of a heart defect. His past history was uneventful, and his physical development quite normal. There was no cyanosis nor dyspnea. Dilated veins were seen in the frontal region, and a marked pattern of veins was seen on both eyelids. He had a left convergent strabismus. General and neurological examination revealed no abnormalities. Routine blood and urine examinations were normal. ESR 6/20. Hematocrite 35%. All the coagulation tests were normal. Chest X-rays showed enlargement of the heart and in lateral projections enlargement of the right and left ventricle. The perihilar pattern was accentuated. Electro-cardiography revealed sinus tachycardia of 135 beats per min., sinistro-atrial P-wave and signs of left heart hypertrophy (Fig. 4).

Cardiac catheterization revealed that the peripheral blood was saturated with oxygen to 94%. Blood pressure in the femoral artery was 95/50 mm of mercury with a mean pressure of 65 mm. There was no evidence of a shunt, and the pressures in the right atrium, right ventricle, and pulmonary artery were normal. The atrial septum was perforated according to the Brockenbrough method, and the left heart was catheterized. pO_2-values and pressure values were normal.

The cardiac output was increased up to twice the normal for the patient's age.

A congenital heart defect had been excluded, but the left heart hypertrophy and considerably increased cardiac output suggested the presence of an arteriovenous shunt. Cerebral angiography confirmed the presence of a huge angioma.

Summary

1. In no case of cerebral angioma did the shunt values correspond to those seen in a hemodynamically active persistent ductus arteriosus. The pulmonary flow volume was at the upper limit of the normal in almost all patients. High O_2-saturation values in the inferior and superior vena cava suggested a hyperkinetic circulation. The O_2-saturation difference between the proximal and distal parts of the jugular vein was so small that it was attributed to the method of examination, and the shunt volume could not be calculated.

2. The circulation time was considerably reduced due to the presence of the arteriovenous short circuit in the blood stream. A correlation between the circulation time and the size of the angioma was found.

3. An expected increase od systolic pressure in the right ventricle
   and pulmonary artery was not found. None of the patients had an
   end-diastolic pressure rise with corresponding increase of the pressure in the right atrium and peripheral venous pressure, suggesting
   myocardial insufficiency.

4. The heart size in all patients was normal. There were no ECG-signs
   of heart overloading.

5. These findings, observed exclusively in adults, contrast with the
   known fact of cardiomegaly due to the presence of a cerebral arteriovenous malformation in children. Cardiomegaly combined with prom-
   inent frontal veins were the only signs of a huge hemispheric angioma.

6. Our investigations suggest that adult patients harboring a cerebral
   arteriovenous malformation, do not have a considerable volume overloading of the heart. Intensive cardiological diagnosis is therefore
   not required. Clinical signs of volume overloading with an increase
   of the heart size and corresponding ECG changes should be an indication for intensive cardiological investigation. The cardiologist
   should be aware that signs of a hyperkinetic blood circulation may
   suggest a cerebral angioma. The neurosurgeon should be aware of the
   possibility of cardiac insufficiency in patients with huge cerebral
   angiomas and should take note of such findings as cardiomegaly and
   corresponding ECG alterations.

Finally, huge angiomas in neonates and children occupy a special position, as they tend to produce early cardiac insufficiency.

R e f e r e n c e s

1. BING, R. J.: The physiology of congenital heart disease. Nelson New
   Loose-Leaf Medicine Vol. V. New York 1949.

2. KEYS, A., SHAPIRO, M. J.: Patency of the ductus arteriosus in adults.
   Amer. Heart J. 25, 158 (1943).

3. EPPINGER, E., BURWELL, S., GROSS, R.: The effects of the patent ductus arteriosus on the circulation. J. Clin. Invest. 20, 127 (1941).

4. DEXTER, L., DOW, G. W., HAYNES, F. W., WHITTENBERGER, L., FERRIS, B.
   G., GOODALE, W. F., HELLEMS, H. K.: Studies of the pulmonary circulation in man at rest. Normal variations and the interrelations between increased pulmonary blood-flow, elevated pulmonary arterial
   pressure, and high "capillary" pressures. J. Clin. Invest. 29, 602
   (1950).

5. LOOGEN, F.: Der pulmonale Hochdruck bei angeborenen Herzfehlern mit
   hohem pulmonalem Stromvolumen. Arch. Kreisl. Forsch. 22, 1 (1958).

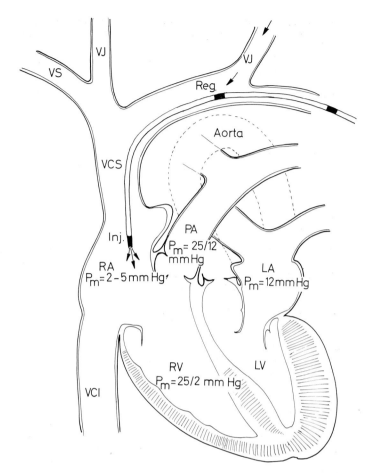

Fig. 1. Position of the catheter at sampling the blood for estimation of O_2-saturation and pressure recording

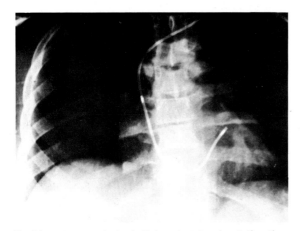

Position of the catheter in R heart and recirculation time in a healthy subject

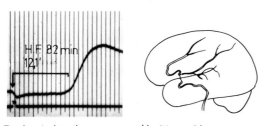

Recirculation time   Healthy subject

Fig. 2. Position of the catheter in R heart and recirculation time in a healthy subject

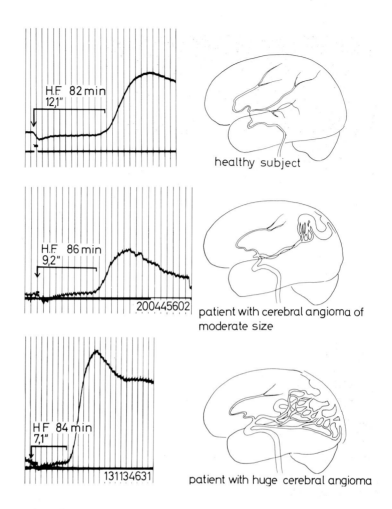

Fig. 3. Recirculation time

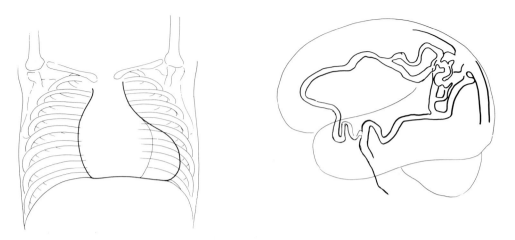

Fig. 4. Cardiomegaly in a 2-years old child with huge parietal angioma
020270101

Discussion on Chapter IV

PIA: Due to functional angiographic examination and the measurement of the general and local cerebral blood flow, the cerebral steal-syndrome due to arteriovenous angiomas has been known for some time. But there is still some uncertainty in its recognition and in anticipating its functional consequences. The introduction of functional tests by which autoregulation and its disturbances can be assessed has led to progress. Intraoperative evaluation of the blood flow, whether with Xenon-techniques, by heat clearance probes or by fluorescence angiography allows a better insight into disturbances of the circulation and may perhaps influence the operative procedure. Modern cardiological examination techniques have allowed the quantitative determination of the effect of the cerebral shunt on the heart and the general circulation. I hope that by means of these techniques the evaluation of compensation and decompensation will become firmer and with it the possibility of the best timing for the operation and an estimation of inoperability.

Many of our guests here have a lot of experience in the direct and indirect measurement of cerebral blood flow. We wondered if we might achieve better results by measuring the cerebral blood flow during the operation, and I think that Dr. Feindel has shown us how important his methods are, not only because of the technique of preparation, but also because of the possibility of avoiding damage to funtionally important areas. Your case with the artery feeding the motor cortex was so impressive that we must adopt your methods, because up till now we have been unable to judge the circulation time intraoperatively.

FEINDEL: We have especially used fluorescein angiography for those angiomas on the surface. I pointed out the advantages in the short presentation, I should also say something about the disadvantages. One disadvantage is that you have a catheter in the internal carotid artery for many hours, just as in selective angiography. We have used a dilute solution of heparin which irrigates the catheter at the rate of 1 cc every 15 or 20 minutes, and we have had no problems with placing the catheter in that way. The catheter placement may take anywhere from 5 minutes to half an hour, depending on how skilful you are when you want to put it in before the operation. Secondly, of course, the great disadvantage of fluorescein angiography is that you do not see the deep vessels. You can only see the surface vessels and this is why I think that intraoperative radiological angiography has a very important role, if one is doing a deep angioma. The third thing is that we still use, from time to time, the injection of a colored dye, not fluorescein, which is particularly useful for identifying deep feeding vessels. It is a very simple procedure if you have the catheter in place to put in

2 cc - we used to use Coomassie blue which is very good, but then it was withdrawn from the market for some reason, but you can use Evan's blue which is perfectly safe and is used by the cardiologists. For example, in a case recently where we had a feeder from the pericallosal artery going down the longitudinal fissure instead of clipping the pericallosal on the normal side, we were able to avoid that by shooting in a little blue dye, and thus we were able to see the abnormal artery very clearly. It is also useful at that stage having clipped the artery, to give another injection to see if you have any back-feeding. So I think this is something that everyone could use and perhaps, in certain circumstances, it would provide more specific information. I just want to make one other point. I believe there is perhaps a great deal of emphasis in discussing the size of a cerebral angioma, on the size of the veins. The veins do not matter a damn, if I may say so. It is the arteries which are important. And in the case we showed up here with the Coomassie Blue showing up that tiny little angioma, the venous phase was really very frightening. It looked as though you would have to take out the whole hemisphere. Now that the radiologists are getting these beautifully detailed and elegant arteriographic pictures, if you analyse the precise arterial input, I think they are quite right to emphasize that you really need a very early phase. Then you often find that what appears to be an inoperable angioma on the mid-phase arteriogram is in fact sometimes quite a simple technical surgical procedure, if you can pick off the feeding arteries. I think this is a most important point to emphasize and you see time and time again in the literature very impressive angiomas, but they are always in the late phase when everything is filled. That has nothing to do with the surgeon except you must know where the surface veins are in order to approach the arteries. And we always tell our radiologists, please call for the film before you inject in order to get the earliest film.

PERRET: Fluorescein angiography apparently helps you a great deal when the arteriovenous malformation is right on the cortex or just below the cortex. Now is there any information that you can obtain about intra or paraventricular malformations with this method? Or is there any other way of finding out, when you have the brain exposed, at what level you should make your incision to come right down on the feeding arteries to a deep-seated a-v malformation?

FEINDEL: We have used small isotope detectors to help us with deep angiomas even though the fluorescein does not show us the vessels. If you get a good shunt peak and then do your arterial occlusion and repeat even the transient time, which is a very quick thing to do, you can identify how much the shunt flow has been reduced. And I think this gives you some guidance as to how much further you have to go.

WÜLLENWEBER: There is nothing to add to the presentation of Dr. Feindel, but with regard to a proven severe cerebral steal syndrome in angiomas, we should think carefully about the indications for operation in the asymptomatic patient. Severely reduced perfusion of the cerebral tissue, particularly in young patients, should lead us to a more active approach to surgery.

PENNING: (to Dr. Feindel) Did you also apply your method to spinal angiomas? I can see a neat combination of your method with that of Dr. Djindjian. One of the nice things of spinal angiomas, of course, is that they are all superficial.

FEINDEL: No, we have not used it in spinal angiomas. It is not quite true that they are all superficial. We have had several cases who came to autopsy in which there was an extension of the angioma into the spinal cord.

PERRET: (to Dr. Feindel) Do you think that a cerebral steal syndrome may still be present even though the patient may have no convulsions nor neurologic deficit? In other words, what are the symptoms that you expect from a cerebral steal?

FEINDEL: This is something I think we must have better documented. It is perfectly true that some of the patients with a cerebral steal, as we all know, have surprisingly little overt neurological deficit. But there is very little in the literature that we have been able to find on the detailed psychological assessment of a patient with a cerebral angioma who has not been operated on, but has been followed over a period of years. There is very little evidence about what happens pre- and postoperatively in a sophisticated psychological way, and I think we need just this information, viz. what is the cerebral steal doing to the brain. We must have much more precise cerebral blood flow measurements over a period of years and pre- and postoperative psychological studies. There is one syndrome which has not been mentioned this morning; at least there is one feature which we think is due to the cerebral steal. When the veins are filled with red arterial blood under pressure, some patients do get papilledema without any focal neurological signs. I think it is a surprising thing that more patients do not have this, but in the last two years we have operated on two patients in whom one of the indications was that they had papilledema. This was of an order that we would not like to see go on. One patient was gradually loosing vision, and the other patient had subjective visual impairment.

KUHLENDAHL: While we are on this topic, I would like to remind you of the investigations of Bernsmeyer and Gottstein 25 years ago, who found a twofold to fourfold increase of the total cerebral blood flow, thus explaining the steal-syndrome. These investigations showed that in addition to the local steal there was an enormous dynamic effect on the general circulation.

PIA: An example of this type of case was presented by Dr. Bauer. It was investigated as a cardiac problem first, and secondarily the diagnosis of a cerebral a-v angioma was arrived at, so maybe cardiologists will send patients to us to find out whether there is a cerebral steal.

Chapter V
Operative Macro- and Microsurgical Treatment

Introduction

H. W. Pia

New surgical techniques have extended the indications for operative treatment of angiomas located in midline structures and in regions of vital and functional importance. The absolute contraindications to treatment of huge cerebral angiomas have also diminished. However, experience is still limited, and there is no uniform approach. Judgement of the natural risk to which an angioma exposes the patient as well as the evaluation of the operative risk and possible consequent neurological deficits is based on multiple, not clearly defined factors among which the subjective opinion and experience of the individual surgeon play an important role. In patients with space occupying lesions the indications and contraindications for surgery are far more clear-cut and objective, whereas in centrally located angiomas it is seldom possible to be so definite unless, maybe, a hematoma causing raised intracranial pressure is found.

The cooperative study showed that an unbiased approach to the analysis of such exceptional and borderline cases is possible. Without trying to diminish the value of such a study one has to admit, however, that statistically significant data do not have much weight in consideration of individual cases.

I would like to illustrate these difficulties with the two following examples, and further cases will be later reported by F. SCHEPELMANN and J. ZIERSKI.

The first case is that of a 38-year-old architect with an angioma located in the left Sylvian fissure and temporal lobe. He had generalized and temporal lobe seizures for three years with attacks of transient complete aphasia occurring for one year. Once the diagnosis was established, a bilateral amytal test suggested that the patient was ambidexterous and a conservative policy was adopted. During the following year the seizures continued. The patient became more irritable, mentally slow, and his working efficiency diminished.

Surgery was performed and the angioma was extirpated totally without difficulty. A few days after the operation he developed the syndrome of a middle cerebral artery thrombosis, which than gradually improved. During the first postoperative year two more generalized fits occurred. When seen 5 years later, he had a distinct amnestic aphasia particularly when under stress. His mental condition was slightly worse than before the operation. He continued to work in his profession, however, in a subordinate capacity. His creativeness and work efficiency remained diminished.

The second example is that of a 31-year-old officer with a cherry-sized angioma within the thalamus upon whom we operated one month after an uncomplicated ventricular hemorrhage. The angioma was extirpated. The residual hematoma in the lateral ventricle was removed. The patient's intention had been to give up his military career, and he did so. At present he is successfully studying philology. His only deficit is a complete homonymous hemianopia.

It seems to me that in both these cases there was a clear indication for surgery. In both of them the operation was successful, but the question must be asked whether possibly another approach or another technique (e.g. embolization) might not have been better in the first case. Surgery was successful, but is the degree of morbidity acceptable?

I have intentionally chosen two not very impressive examples, and I have not mentioned patients with huge angiomas, lethal complications, or major deficits, in order to emphasize the delicate and difficult assessment of the risk for each individual patient and to point out the particular responsibility we carry in just such cases.

I do hope that the following reports about the possibilities and limitations of conventional and microsurgical methods of treatment of hitherto unapproachable malformations will enable us to define better the indications and contraindications for surgery.

Extensive Cerebellar Arteriovenous Malformations

Z. KUNC

Introduction

The surgery of arteriovenous malformations (AVM) has made considerable progress since its early beginnings. Its trend has been all the time to advance beyond what had been hitherto the limits of operability. Surgical success in so called inoperable cases has been reported of late. Deeply located and extensive AVM still remain a rather difficult problem and some of those in the cerebellum are amongst them. Small AVM on the posterior cerebellar surface may be removed easily (1, 2). Large AVM, however, are quite a problem (3), their resection being hazardous (4). In most cases they are considered to be inoperable (5, 6). More than 50 radically treated cerebellar cases have been reported so far but large and deeply-sited lesions are very rare (8, 1, 3, 2, 5, 4, 9), with a very high rate of mortality (4). Having a frequency of 5 to 20% (3, 7), cerebellar AVM deserve special attention.

Material and Methods

Over a period of 20 years intracranial AVM have been diagnosed at the Clinic of Neurosurgery in Prague in 157 patients, in 10 of them (6.4%) in the cerebellum. Seven of these 10 patients were males, 3 females. The age of the patients at the onset of symptomatology was: 13, 16, 23, 27, 28, 29, 33, 44, 44, and 57 years.

All these 10 patients were examined by serial vertebral angiography.

The AVM were of very large volume, amounting to $10.45cm^3$ - $65.2cm^3$, with only one of $1.46cm^3$. Their distribution is shown in Table 1.

Four AVMs were mainly supplied by the superior cerebellar artery (Figs. 1, 2). The basal AVM was fed from the posterior inferior and anterior inferior cerebellar arteries and also from the superior cerebellar artery (Fig. 3). The hemisphere AVM was not only supplied from all the cerebellar arteries on the same side, but also partly from the vessels of the opposite side from the occipital artery and from the internal carotid system. The lesion in the lower vermis was fed by the inferior cerebellar arteries only. The supply to the AVM near the confluence of the sinuses was via the tentorial vessels from both carotid arteries, via branches of both vertebral arteries and via both occipital arteries The AVM in the foramen magnum was fed from the vertebral artery.

Table 1. Surgical results

Distribution	Number of cases	Ligation and Coagulation	Ligation alone	Results excellent	good
Anterior and superior part of the right hemisphere	4	2	2	2	2
Base of the left hemisphere	1	1	-	1	-
Entire right hemisphere and vermis	1	-	-	-	-
Midline - vermis	3	1	-	1	-
Left hemisphere with extracranial extension	1	-	1	-	1
Total	10	4	3	4	3

The intracerebellar malformation with extracranial extension obtained blood from the external carotid and the vertebral arteries. The veins draining the AVM led to various sinuses of the posterior fossa and in four cases also to the great vein of Galen (Fig. 1). The shunt of the AVM located at the level of the confluence of the sinuses reversed the blood flow in the straight and sagittal sinuses and in the internal and superior cerebral veins due to thrombosis of both transverse sinuses.

In 6 patients the AVM manifested itself by subarachnoid bleeding with recurrence in two at intervals of 4 and 14 years respectively. In two instances the hemorrhage was serious (Fig. 1) with unconsciousness, associated once with epileptic seizures and mental disorientation. In 3 patients after bleeding there were symptoms of cerebellar dysfunction, in one cerebellar dysarthria, in one diplopia and in two mild hemiparesis. In one patient the hemorrhage resulted in raised intracranial pressure with blurred vision, this grave condition ending in decortication and death.

In 4 patients the evolution of the clinical picture was chronic. One patient suffered from headaches in the suboccipital region for 5 years with cerebellar symptoms. In one patient with a similar headache there was the sudden appearance of a neocerebellar syndrome with diplopia and nystagmus (Fig. 3).Unusual manifestations of an AVM were intermittent visual field defects, their frequency increasing under physical strain (Fig. 2). One patient suffered from headaches, an intracranial bruit and grand mal epilepsy.

R e s u l t s

No treatment was given to three patients. One of them had an AVM occupying the entire hemisphere, but mild symptoms. One patient was in poor general condition. The third patient, with the AVM at the level of the confluence of the sinuses, died from a recurrent hemorrhage.

Seven patients were operated upon, 4 by a temporal approach and incision of the tentorium, 2 suboccipitally, and one by both routes in a two-stage procedure (Fig. 3). In 4 patients, occlusion of the main artery of supply and of some further vessels, together with as radical a coagulation of the AVM as possible was performed. In 3 patients the procedure was confined to occlusion of the main feeding artery only. In 2 cases the operation was radical; it was almost radical in 1 case; and in 4 cases the malformation was significantly reduced. The arteriovenous shunt decreased after the palliative procedures to such an extent that the vertebral and basilar arteries diminished in diameter.

The clinical results were quite satisfactory (Table 1). The patients who were evaluated as excellent were either without any symptoms or with a mild residual deficit; they became fully active again. The results were considered to be only good in those patients in whom the procedure was followed by the development of fresh symptoms. One patient developed burning paresthesia in half the face and in the extremities of the same side four months after the operation (Fig. 1). The intracranial bruit disappeared in one patient, but the headaches increased. In one patient there appeared a homonymous field defect, attacks of depressions, and bouts of falling asleep. He died 3 years later of brain oedema after a car accident.

Two patients who were surgically treated have now been alive for 7 years, one for 12 years, and two for almost 3 years.

Discussion

The clinical symptoms of cerebellar AVM are well known. Our experiences are in accord with what has been published (3, 4). Serial vertebral angiography as generally used has solved all diagnostic problems. An unusual clinical observation from our experience is that a strong arteriovenous shunt from the cerebellar arteries may provoke a steal syndrome even in the cerebral vascular bed. The paroxysmal hemianopia in one of our patients may thus be explained. The posterior cerebral artery on the side of the malformation was opacified by the contrast medium only on the postoperative angiogram (Fig. 2).

The indications for a surgical attack on a cerebellar AVM should comprise not only the extent of the symptomatology, but also the uncertain future for a patient with this type of lesion (9). Both the hemorrhage and the long-term harmful effects of an arteriovenous shunt on the surrounding nervous tissue may cause grave disability and even death. Surgery is always indicated if the AVM has bled (3). With chronic syndromes, an expectant attitude may be adopted . Extensive and deeply sited lesions should be judged individually from all aspects (9). It should be borne in mind that the approach to some sites is rather intricate. This is where the principle that the procedure can not be stopped half way applies with more than usual force. A hemorrhage in the depths of the posterior fossa could be most dramatic. Malformations of this type may not be, however, surgically contraindicated. Often they are chiefly supplied by one or two main arteries with the other tributaries being small collaterals. This does not mean that occlusion of the supplying artery alone could eliminate the AVM from the circulation. However it suffices for the most part to prevent further bleeding and to improve the symptoms. A significant decrease of the arteriovenous shunt is well shown by the delayed and greatly decreased filling of the AVM which occurs only in the capillary phase and by the decrease in diameter of the vertebral and basilar arteries (Fig. 2). There is no dispute that the object of the operation should be the complete elimination of the AVM from circulation. Resection is the best method (1), but in some cases it can not be realized (3), and may be rather hazardous (4). Occlusion of the feeding arteries along with coagulation of the AVM is advised as being effective and applicable in almost any cerebellar AVM, yet with a minimum of risk. In our experience this procedure has not been the cause of death nor of any grave disability in spite of the fact that all the lesions were very large.

A subtemporal transtentorial approach proved to be good in cases where the AVM was sited anteriorly or superiorly. This approach is not hindered by large draining veins, whereas the primary occlusion of them necessary in the suboccipital approach is dangerous in extensive lesions because of the increased pressure inside them and the possibility of rupture.

Both these approaches should be combined if the malformations are very large (4).

S u m m a r y

Cerebellar AVM was diagnosed in 10 patients. In six of them the lesions were very large varying from 10.45 cm^3 to 65.2 cm^3. 2 replaced an entire hemisphere and one extended extracranially in addition. Four patients were operated on by a subtemporal transtentorial approach, 2 by a suboccipital approach and one by both. In 3, only occlusion of the supplying artery was carried out but in 4 coagulation of the AVM was also performed. The operation was radical in 2 cases, almost radical in 1 and with a significantly reduced malformation in 4. Nobody died. The results were excellent in 4 and good in 3 patients.

A c k n o w l e d g e m e n t

The author express many thanks to Dr. J. Bret for angiographic examinations and to Mr. L. Slavík for his photographic work.

R e f e r e n c e s

1. POOL, J. L., POTTS, D. G.: Aneurysms and arteriovenous anomalies of the brain. Diagnosis and treatment. New York: Hoeber 1965.

2. MORELLO, G.: Some aspects of the surgery of cerebral arteriovenous angiomas. Third Europ. Congr. Neurosurg. Excerpta Med. (Amsterdam) 139, 31-32 (1967).

3. LAINE, E., GALIBERT, P.: Anévrysmes artério-veineux et cirsoides de la fosse postérieure. Rev. Neurol. 115, 276-288 (1966).

4. VERBIEST, H.: Arteriovenous aneurysms of the posterior fossa. In: Luyendijk, W. (ed.): Cerebral circulation, p. 383-396. Amsterdam-London-New York: Elsevier 1968.

5. KRAYENBÜHL, H., YASARGIL, M. G.: Das Hirnaneurysma. Docum. Geigy. Series chir. Basle 1968.

6. WAPPENSCHMIDT, J., GROTE, W., HOLBACH, K. H.: Diagnosis and therapy of arteriovenous malformations shown by vertebral angiography. In: Luyendijk, W. (ed.): Cerebral Circulation, p. 411-418. Amsterdam-London-New York: Elsevier 1968.

7. PERRET, G., NISHIOKA, H.: Arteriovenous malformations (an analysis of 545 cases of cranio-cerebral arteriovenous malformations and fistulas). J. Neurosurgery. 25, 467-490 (1966).

8. SCHULTZ, E. C., HUSTON, W. A.: Arteriovenous aneurysm of the posterior fossa in an infant. Report of a case. J. Neurosurgery. 13, 211-214 (1965).

9. KUNC, Z.: Arteriovenózní malformace mozku (Arteriovenous malformations of the brain, in Czech.) Čas. lék. čes. 110, 897-903 (1971).

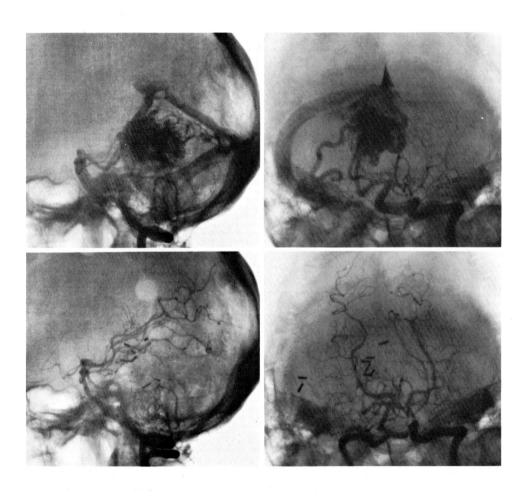

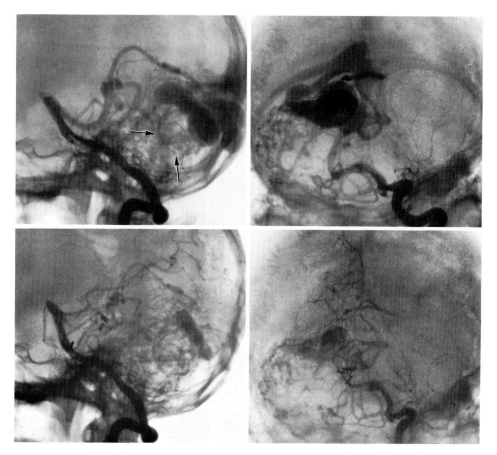

Fig. 2. Case 2. A man aged 23 years. Intermittent defects in the right half of the visual field. <u>Vertebral angiogram</u>. AVM supplied from the superior cerebellar artery. Calcification indicated by arrows (arrowhead). Posterior cerebral artery not filled. Drainage into the confluence of the sinuses. <u>Control</u> after ligature of the superior cerebellar artery by subtemporal approach. AVM is only partly filled. Posterior cerebral artery has again become visible. Redcution of the diameter of the vertebral and basilar arteries. The attacks of visual field defects ceased

◀ Fig. 1. Case 1. A man aged 49 years. Two subarachnoid hemorrhages; palaeo- and neo-cerebellar syndrome; hemiparesis. <u>Vertebral angiogram</u>. AVM chiefly supplied from the superior cerebellar artery and drained through the great vein of Galen. <u>Control</u> after ligature of the superior cerebellar artery and coagulation of the AVM by a subtemporal and transtentorial approach. Mild cerebellar symptoms remained. A burning feeling appeared in the left hand and in the face

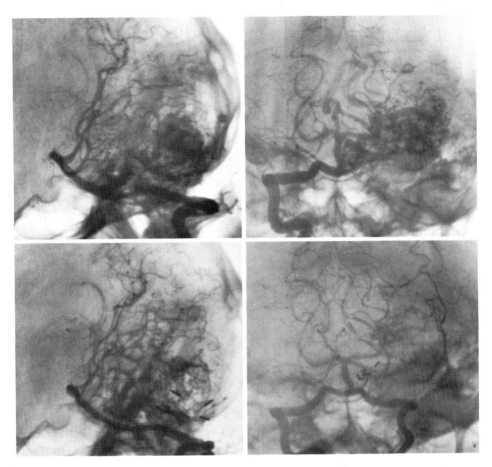

Fig. 3. Case 3. A man aged 30 years. Suboccipital headache, diplopia, nystagmus, left neocerebellar syndrome.
Vertebral angiogram. AVM fed mainly by the posterior inferior and anterior inferior cerebellar arteries and by the superior cerebellar artery. Drainage into the confluence of the sinuses and great vein of Galen. Control after ligatures of the main feeding arteries and coagulation of the AVM in two stages. AVM still persists in part. The patient has now been without any neurological deficit and any complaint for 7 years

Macro- and Microsurgery of Central Angiomas

K.-A. Bushe, J. Bockhorn and E. R. Schäfer

Introduction

In an unselected series of cases at the University Neurosurgical Clinic of Göttingen we have seen 56 angioma cases, 20 of which were located in or near the midline of the brain.

17 of these 20 patients were treated surgically, 3 patients were excluded from surgical treatment.

Material and Methods

Classification of angiomas with regrad to the indication for and techniques of surgery.

Following HENDERSON (1) and MORELLO (2) we group angiomas according to their size:

1. Small angiomas with a diameter of less than 2 cm.

2. Medium Size angiomas with a diameter between 2 and 6 cm.

3. Large angiomas with a diameter of more than 6 cm.

The most common symptoms are epileptic seizures, hemorrhage, or a combination of both. Reviewing the cases of the Göttingen Neurosurgical Clinic, we found that seizures are more common with angiomas of the parietal lobe, whereas angiomas of the frontal, temporal or occipital lobes present with hemorrhages as well as seizures. The reason that angiomas of the parietal lobe bleed only rarely may be found in the fact that seizures direct attention to the lesion prior to its bleeding. In our experience, we can state that angiomas of the midline, especially of the basal ganglia, the midbrain and the cerebellum in general do not cause seizures, and the first indication of their presence is a hemorrhage.

As a second result of our study, we found that small angiomas bleed far more often than larger ones and the intracerebral clot itself is relatively extensive in small angiomas.

In answer to the question, whether macro- or microsurgical methods should be employed, the principle, judging from our experience, should be that all angiomas should be operated upon under the microscope. The reasons for this statement have been published before and need no repetition. In small angiomas, especially in cases where the angioma lies deep and has to be approached through a narrow field, the help of an operating microscope due to the better lighting and the magnification is self-evident. In medium size angiomas one has - according to the nature and size of the angioma - to choose between the microscope and surgical telescopes, the latter combined with a good headlight. In large and widespread angiomas the operating microscope was found to be inconvenient and surgical telescopes were preferred.

Our observations on angiomas located in different midline sites will now be reported.

6 arteriovenous angiomas were located in the interhemispheric fissure, totally or partly involving the corpus callosum. Three of these angiomas were excluded from our surgical series because it was feared that surgery might result in death or severe neurological damage. Of the remaining angiomas in this location one was removed with good results and in two other cases the feeding vessels were ligated. In one of these latter cases the angiographic follow-up showed a total elimination of the angioma with good post-operative results. On the other hand we lost a two year old child after ligature because of diffuse, intractable gastric bleeding. Out of our cases these two are the only ones in which we saw an indication for ligating the feeding vessels.

Para- and intraventricular angiomas are regarded as inoperable by a number of authors for they cause considerable technical problems during surgery.

We have seen 8 angiomas in this location. Prior to surgery, angiomas located at the trigone or in the temporal horn require vertebral as well as carotid angiography. One case may be reported in support of this recommendation which was first made many years ago: This was a 40-year-old woman, who during childhood had two episodes of intracranial bleeding. During pregnancy recurrent bleeding occurred. Carotid angiography, carried out after delivery, demonstrated an angioma of the posterior part of the temporal lobe, presumably located intraventricularly. The arrangement of the abnormal feeding vessels tempted one to ligate them and this caused no problems. Control carotid angiography led to the false conclusion that the angioma had been totally eliminated. Nevertheless vertebral angiography still demonstrated filling of the angioma. At a second operation the widespread intraventricular angioma was totally removed.

As a result of this experience we now examine preoperatively both vascular trees in all angiomas of this region. All of these 8 intraventricular angiomas were removed and 6 showed very good results. We lost two patients, both of whom had been admitted to the hospital as emergencies with ventricular tamponade following intraventricular bleeding.

Angiomas of the basal ganglia and the midbrain come rarely to surgery and will be even more rarely totally removed (3). To follow the advice, frequently given, to ligate only the feeding vessels does not give satisfactory results, for, in our experience, angiomas may also be fed by other vessels which cannot be demonstrated by angiography.

We have seen two patients with angiomas situated in the basal ganglia subependymal to the trigone (4).

In a six-year-old boy we first tried to approach the angioma transventricularly in the usual way. In spite of definite angiographic localisation and close inspection during surgery we were unable to find the angioma owing to its site, hidden beneath the ependyma. To avoid further damage from surgical trauma, we stopped the procedure.

At a second operation we approached the dome of the angioma stereotactically and removed it in the usual manner transventricularly, using the operating microscope. Though the thalamo-striate vein had to be clipped, the postoperative course was without further complication. The boy showed no residual signs from the hemorrhage and the removal.

In a 19-year-old female patient we were able to remove an angioma localized in the same area, using the experience gained from the above-mentioned case. The angioma was approached stereotactically and removed by a transventricular approach using the operating microscope.

The extirpation was much more difficult in this second case than in the six-year-old boy, for the ventricles were fairly small. The postoperative course was without complication except for some extrapyramidal impairment.

In the meantime the patient had a normal pregnancy and gave birth to a healthy child.

The first and only symptom in both cases was an intraventricular hemorrhage.

R e s u l t s

Altogether we have operated on 46 angiomas (Table 1), 4 of these with fatal results, three of which were localized near the midline of the brain. This is a mortality rate of 8.7%. In 3 of the patients with a fatal result we had to start operating against a background of progressive hemorrhage or ventricular tamponade. The fourth of the patients was a 2-year-old child who died of uncontrollable gastric hemorrhage.

Excluding the 3 above-mentioned fatalities who were admitted to the clinic deeply comatose and in whom the fatal result was due to the spontaneous bleeding itself and not to the surgery, a total mortality rate of 2.3% was found.

Considering the angiomas of the midline, we operated on 17 out of 20 patients with 3 fatal results. This is a mortality rate of 17.6%. Excluding the above-mentiones 2 cases who had to be operated on in the stage of the acute hemorrhage, we find a mortality rate of 6.6% after surgery for angiomas of the midline.

Table 1. Distribution of angiomas

Location of angiomas	Number of cases	Total extirpation	Lig. of feeding artery	Removal of hemorrh.	No operation	Results Excellent or good	Deficits mild	severe	Autopsy
1. Cerebral									
a) important area	15	15				12	2	1	
b) polar angioma	15	15				15			
2. Midline angioma	8	2	3		3	3	1		1 (gastric hemorrhage)
3. Ventricular and paraventr. angioma	8	8				6			2 (ventric. hemorrhage)
4. Multiple angioma	1	1				1			
5. Angioma of basal ganglia	2	2				1	1		
6. Cerebellar angioma	2	2				1	1 (Loc. brachia conjunctiva)		
7. Spongeous, inop. angioma	4			1	3				1 (cerebral hemorrhage)
8. Intra- and extra-cranial angioma	2	1	1			2			
Total	57	46	4	1	6	41	5	1	4

Discussion

Finally we want to stress the important points of this particular subject:

We agree with the majority of other authors that all angiomas with a cerebral steal syndrome and angiomas that continue to bleed should be totally removed as far as operative techniques allow this to be done without producing lasting damage. This certainly includes all angiomas of the midline (5, 6, 7, 8, 9). Angiomas with continuing hemorrhage or those with ventricular tamponade should be excluded from surgery. Even when progressive deterioration follows recurrent bleeding, an attempt at operation will not improve the patient's chances.

As this synopsis has proved, however, angiomas of the midline cannot be considered as inoperable. With certain surgical and technical aids such as the stereotactic approach, the use of the operating microscope, and intraoperative induced hypotension, ventricular and paraventricular angiomas as well as angiomas of the basal ganglia and the cerebellum have to be considered for operation.

The mortality rate after surgical intervention is not prohibitively high.

Summary

Angiomas of the midline cannot be considered as inoperable. With certain surgical and technical aids ventricular and paraventricular angiomas as well as angiomas of the basal ganglia and the cerebellum have to be considered for operation. Considering the angiomas of the midline we operated upon 17 out of 20 patients.

References

1. HENDERSON, W. R., GOMEZ, R. L.: Natural history of cerebral angiomas. Brit. med. J. 4, 571-574 (1967).

2. MORELLO, G., BORGHI, G. P.: Central angiomas. Acta neurochir. (Wien) 135-155 (1973).

3. RIECHERT, T., MUNDINGER, F.: Combined stereotaxic operation for treatment of deepseated angiomas and aneurysms. J. Neurosurgery 21, 358-363 (1964).

4. BUSHE, K.-A., PETERSON, E., SCHÄFER, E. R.: Surgical interventions for arterio-venous angiomas in functionally important regions and in case of spreading within the area of the ventricular system of the basal ganglia. In: Fusek, I., Kunc, Z. (eds.): Present Limits of Neurosurgery. Proceedings of the fourth European Congress of Neurosurgery. Avicenum. Prague: Czechoslovak Medical Press 1972.

5. BUSHE, K.-A.: Behandlung von Gefäßprozessen des Zentralnervensystems unter besonderer Berücksichtigung mikrochirurgischer Methoden. Berichte der Physikalisch-Medizinischen Gesellschaft zu Würzburg 81, 133-144 (1973).

6. BUSHE, K.-A.: Möglichkeiten einer operativen Behandlung intracranieller Gefäßanomalien und Gefäßverschlüsse. Verh. Dtsch. Ges. Kreislaufforschung Bd. 39, 73-79 (1973).

7. BARTAL, A. D.: Excision of bleeding paraventricular arteriovenous malformations. Excerpta Medica International Congress Series No 193 (1969).

8. BARTAL, A. D., YAKEL, M.: Total excision of arteriovenous malformation of the corpus callosum. J. Neurosurgery XXXIII, 95-99 (1970).

9. MILHORAT, T. H.: Excision of a cirsoid arteriovenous malformation of the corpus callosum in a 16-year-old boy. J. Neurosurgery, XXXIII, 339-344 (1970).

Stereotactic Treatment of Central Angiomas

T. RIECHERT

In order to determine the operability of an angioma we are bound essentially to consider 3 points:

1. a location in the brain stem, especially in mid-line structures;

2. its situation in the immediate neighbourhood of functionally important brain centers;

3. and independently of these first 2 points whether the angioma is of extraordinary size and what are its feeding vessels.

In a subsequent description of a new method of localization and surgery of vascular malformations, I want to discuss principally and in detail the two first points, and to underline their importance by giving some examples of patients on whom we have operated.

Using this method we have operated on deep-seated small angiomas which for the most part were located subcortically in the region of the III. ventricle or the basal ganglia, and chiefly in the thalamus or neighbouring structures. We know that it is relatively small vascular tumors that are likely to cause recurrent hemorrhages. Considering their proximity to the ventricles, the possiblity of a tamponade of the ventricles and subsequent states of prolonged unconsciousness seems likely. For these reasons it is important to extirpate these angiomas. Except in 2 cases, we have chosen extirpation, regarding the ligature of the feeding vessels merely as an emergency procedure.

Typically an open operation on a deep-seated angioma necessitates a relatively large resection of cerebral cortex and of subcortical structures or an incision in the corpus callosum before the angioma is extirpated. This method faces the following problems:

1. Functional deficits are easily caused by the relatively large resection of cortex and white matter.

2. In the depth of brain, in the region of the basal ganglia, the anatomical orientation as well as the identification of the feeding vessels becomes more and more difficult.

Numerous cases have been published where postoperative angiography has shown that only part of the feeding vessels or of the angioma had been resected. In order to facilitate orientation, for the most part the shortest and most direct way to resect the malformation has been preferred, but this method often leads to functional deficits. These facts have contributed to the opinion that part of these deep-seated tumors seemed to be inoperable, and that the results were hardly encouraging.

A new and possible method of treatment of these deep-seated angiomas was provided by the stereotactic method. The probe could reach the angioma with great precision without resection of any cortex. By special methods it was now possible to treat the angioma with the help of the probe, which was constructed as a magnet, as an electrode or as special clip-holding forceps (1).

We have not used this method because an operation in the depths of the brain on a malformation consisting only of vessels did not seem advisable without direct visual control.

Favourable results might be anticipated from a procedure combining the typical open surgery and the stereotactic method. This method seemed promising because it had been performed some years before (2) in order to expose deep-seated foreign bodies. Recently it has been used by other authors with favourable results. The same situation applies in angiomas. By the usual large exposure of the dura a good field of vision is guaranteed. We can operate under direct visual control, and we can alter the approach to the angioma during the operation. The use of the target apparatus and the probe renders it possible to reach the angioma with great reliability. The exposure of the angioma is carried out under direct visual control along the probe. Thus a big resection of the cortex and of subcortical tissue is not necessary.

If this method of operation is used, we avoid the difficulties mentioned above:

1. the functional deficits caused by resection of brain tissue, and

2. the uncertainty in localizing the angioma and its feeding vessels.

A new principle is also used in the localization of these angiomas: As we have seen, in stereotactic surgery the anatomical localization of the subcortical structures is only possible with the help of an encephalogram. Stereotactic operations in the region of the basal ganglia, e.g. in extrapyramidal motor disturbances, require exact anatomical analysis of the structures in which we wish to place lesions in order to avoid secondary damage. In cases of malformations the same precision should be reached. Thus it is important operating on angiomas in this neighbourhood to avoid the laterally situated structures by working in the region of the ventrocaudal thalamus in order not to injure the essential pyramidal fibers. Our experience with these angiomas, which have been localized precisely on X-ray has shown that, in these particular cases, the pure neurological findings may be misleading with respect to the anatomical relations of these angiomas. The operations on the angiomas were carried out with our target apparatus which I constructed with WOLFF (3), and refined with MUNDINGER (4). Using this apparatus we have performed more than 5000 operations up to the present.

The first publication of angiomas operated on by us appeared in 1962 (5), other summaries of further cases were published together with MUNDINGER in 1964 (6) and KRAINICK 1973 (7).

The technique is as follows. In the angiogram we determine whether the angioma in question is suitable for the procedure (Figs. 1, 2). Then follows the mathematical correction of the magnification in the X-ray pictures. The angioma and its feeding vessels are transferred to the encephalogram. Now we have to determine the distance of the angioma from the base line (Foramen of Monro - posterior commissure) in the lateral X-ray, and the distance of the angioma from the midline in the AP-picture. With the help of a phantom brain or atlas we have to determine the anatomical localization of the angioma and its relation to the surrounding structures of the brain, and we have to compare it with the neurological findings. On the day of operation the basal ring of the target apparatus is fixed to the patient's skull, the target point is transferred to the corresponding radiograph, and the electrode is focussed on the target point in the phantom apparatus. Then the trepanation of the skull is performed, and after the exposure of the dura the probe is introduced (Fig. 3). To begin with the probe is not yet inserted to the full depth in order to avoid a lesion of the angioma. The point at which the probe is inserted is selected so as to minimize the neurological deficit. In this manner we can aim consecutively at several structures, e.g. feeding vessels and the angioma itself. Then follows the exposure along the line of the probe under the operating microscope after resecting a small piece of brain tissue (Fig. 4). The exposure of a midline tumor can be made not only interhemispherically, but also by an approach through a hemisphere. Since no topographical errors can occur with this procedure, the length of the approach does not matter. The use of an operating microscope is necessary in these cases, if only for the illumination of the operation zone in the depth of the brain. It is also important to be able to change the approach. During the operation we can decide if the angioma has been extirpated completely on the basis of the exact position of the clips (Figs. 5, 6).

Up till now we have operated on 18 patients with vascular malformations in the region of the basal ganglia and the III. ventricle using the combined open-stereotactic method. In all cases, with one exception, one or more hemorrhages had preceded the surgical intervention. Late results have been evaluated in 14 patients (8). There were no deaths in our 18 patients in the immediate postoperative period. One of our patients suffered a fatal hemorrhage 23 days after operation while walking up and down, waiting for an X-ray picture in the radiological department. He suffered from a thalamic syndrome with a thalamic hand and hemihypesthesia caused by an angioma in the right ventrocaudal thalamus. The symptoms appeared after a spontaneous hemorrhage beginning with paresthesia in the left hand. After the operation the thalamic syndrome had disappeared. Another patient had an angioma in the region of the right oral basal ganglia. 2 1/2 years after operation he showed increasing drowsiness. Death followed with the signs of broncho-pneumonia. The post-mortem examination showed, contrary to our expectations, no fresh hemorrhage but a progressive gliosis and porencephaly in the region of the basal ganglia. Among the 12 surviving patients, 8 returned to their occupations full-time or part-time. Among 4 patients operated on recently, the neurological disturbances of 2 have improved considerably. These 4 patients are not yet recorded in our statistics. One of these patients could return to his usual activities 6 months after the operation, and the same result can be expected in the other cases. Our experience shows that in the main all those patients remained incapacitated, who preoperatively manifested serious neurological deficits, resulting from previous hemorrhages.

Finally I want to mention the experience of other authors who applied the stereotactic method to cases of vascular malformations. GUIOT (9) performed the exposure of an angioma and of an aneurysm along the puncture channel of a flexible probe after localizing the lesion stereotactically. Recently ALKSNE, FINGERHUT, and RAND (10) applied the stereotactic method to cure deep-seated aneurysms with the help of artificially produced thrombosis. They introduced to the neighbourhood of the aneurysm a magnet in the shape of a probe. After injection of very fine particles of iron into the carotid artery and into the aneurysm, respectively, these iron particles were arrested in the aneurysm and caused a thrombosis.

Summing up, we can say that the described method of combined open stereotactic operation does not mean the replacement of the standard methods used until now.

It is, however, an advance in the treatment of vascular malformations in the subcortex, especially in the basal ganglia, and in cerebral regions of great functional importance.

S u m m a r y

For the extirpation of subcortical angiomas, especially in the region of the basal ganglia, a new method of operation has been devised: a combination of the stereotactic method with a classical craniotomy, associated with a new procedure for localizing the angioma. The author reports on 18 patients operated on with the described method.

R e f e r e n c e s

1. ALKSNE, J. F., FINGERHUT, A., RAND, R.: Magnetically controlled metallic thrombosis of intracranial aneurysms. Surgery St. Louis 60, 212-218 (1966).

2. RIECHERT, T.: Die Entfernung von tiefsitzenden Hirnstecksplittern mit Hilfe des stereotaktischen Operationsverfahrens. Zbl. Neurochir. 15, 159-164 (1955).

3. RIECHERT, T., WOLFF, M.: Über ein neues Zielgerät zur intrakraniellen elektrischen Ableitung und Ausschaltung. Arch. Psychiatr. 186, 225-230 (1951).

4. RIECHERT, T., MUNDINGER, F.: Beschreibung und Anwendung eines Zielgerätes für stereotaktische Hirnoperationen (II. Modell). Acta neurochir., Wien, Suppl. III, 308-337 (1955).

5. RIECHERT, T.: Eine neue Methode zur Behandlung bisher inoperabler arterio-venöser Angiome: Die Operation auf stereotaktischem Wege. "Medical Congress" Prag, 12.-17.11.1962 anläßlich der Hundertjahrfeier der Tschechischen Medizinischen Gesellschaft.

6. RIECHERT, T., MUNDINGER, F.: Combined stereotaxic operation for treatment of deep-seated angiomas and aneurysms. J. Neurosurg., Springfield 21, 358-363 (1964).

7. KRAINICK, J.-U.: Kombiniert offen-stereotaktische Operationen bei Angiomen im Bereich der Stammganglien. III. Internationales Symposium über die Diagnostik und Therapie der spontanen Subarachnoidalblutung, Graz, 28.-30.6.1973.

8. SCHULZE, A. D.: Das kombinierte offen-stereotaktische Operationsverfahren zur Behandlung von subcortikalen arteriovenösen Angiomen und Aneurysmen und seine Ergebnisse. Inaugural-Dissertation Freiburg i. Br. (1972).

9. GUIOT, G., ROUGERIE, J., SACHS, M., HERZOG, E., MOLINA, P.: Repérage stéréotaxique de malformations vasculaires profondes intracérébrales. La Semaine des Hôpitaux 36, 1134-1143 (1960).

10. (see ref. 1.).

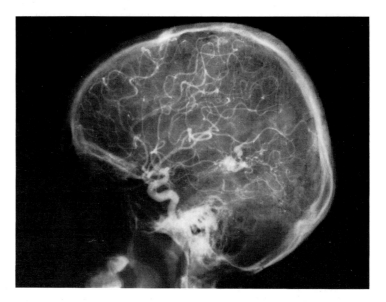

Fig. 1. Deep-seated angioma. Right sided angiography. Symptoms: Paralysis of the nervus oculomotorius and hemiplegia alternans (Weber's syndrome)

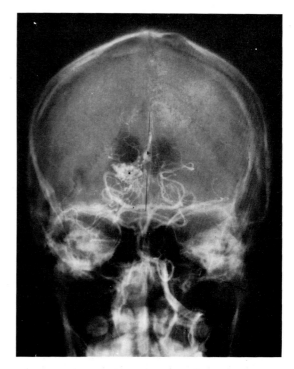

Fig. 2. Angiography of the same case. a. p. picture

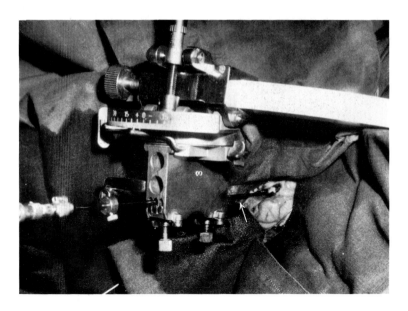

Fig. 3. Operation-picture. Introduction of the probe for the cortical resection

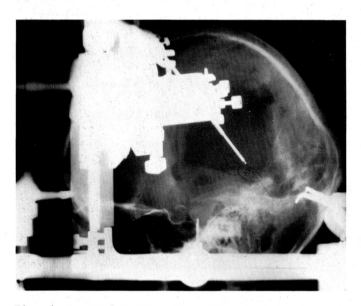

Fig. 4. Lateral X-ray. The probe is introduced to the angioma (see Figs. 1, 2)

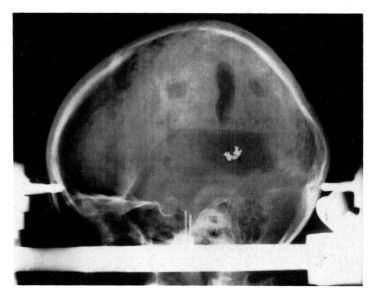

Fig. 5. Intraoperative X-ray picture after clipping of the angioma. The position of the clips corresponds to the extirpated angioma

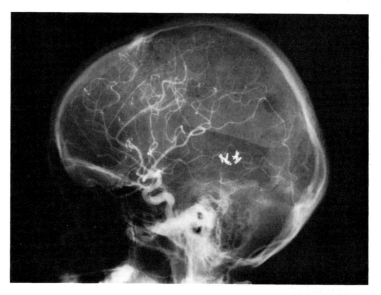

Fig. 6. X-ray check-up: Angiography of the same case. The angioma was extirpated completely, which can also be shown in the other angiographic phases. The clips are situated in the position of the extirpated vascular malformation

Angiomas of Cerebellum and Brain Stem

C. LAPRAS

Since the first successful excision of a cerebellar angioma accomplished
by OLIVECRONA and RIIVES in 1948 (1), an increasing number have been
reported (2, 3, 4, 5, 6, 7, 8). Angiomas of the cerebellum and brain
stem are fed by the vertebro-basilar system. However distal angiomas
of the posterior cerebral artery must be excluded because they belong
to the supra-tentorial angiomas, and their therapeutic problems are
very different. The distal angiomas of the posterior choroidal artery
must also be excluded (thalamic or intra-ventricular angiomas). But it
seems necessary to keep in this study angiomas fed by proximal branches
of the posterior choroidal artery and small branches of the first portion of the posterior cerebral artery or mesencephalic artery (quadrigeminal plates and mesencephalic angiomas, and aneurysms of the vein
of Galen).

The first classification was suggested by V. LOGUE (3) and he contrast-
ed cerebellar angiomas with brain stem angiomas. VERBIEST (6) describes
two types: intra-parenchymatous in the cerebellum and the brain stem,
and arachnoidian (vein of Galen and cerebello-pontine angle). GALIBERT
differentiated two anatomical forms: proximal and distal arteriovenous
aneurysms. For ourselves we keep to the classification of LOGUE and
MONCKTON but in addition divide the brain-stem angiomas into different
anatomical groups thus:

- cerebellar angiomas (cerebellum and vermis).
- brain stem angiomas: diffuse (cerebellum; cervical spinal cord; hypothalamus; Blanc-Bonnet-Dechaume syndrome).
  localised (quadrigeminal plate; mesencephalic; posterior-choroidal
  artery; aneurysm of the vein of Galen; cerebello-pontine angle).

Our study is based on 19 cases:

 5 cases of cerebellar angiomas
14 cases of brain stem angiomas: 2 diffuse; 2 quadrigeminal plate; 2
mesencephalic; 3 proximal posterior-choroidal artery; 4 aneurysms of
the vein of Galen; 1 cerebello-pontine angle).

These different anatomical forms can present with ischemic or hemorrhagic symptoms. Subarachnoid hemorrhage is not restricted to cerebellar angiomas, and we noted it in three cases of brain stem angiomas.
The occurrence of an intracerebellar hematoma is very common from cerebellar angiomas, but it can also complicate brain stem angiomas (two
personal cases). Spontaneous intracerebellar hematomas due to a small
peripheral angioma found at surgery and not shown by angiography have
been reported by many authors (9, 10, 11, 12, 13, 14). We found the

same in one case but we excluded from this study another case of spontaneous intracerebellar hematoma where it was impossible to discover the cause of the bleeding.

Obstructive hydrocephalus is a symptom commonly noted. It can be due to the compression from an asymptomatic cerebellar hematoma. It is more often observed during compression of the Aqueduct of Sylvius by a circumpeduncular angioma or a dilated vein of Galen. Hydrocephalus was noted in our 4 cases of aneurysms of vein of Galen. The frequency of congenital or secondary heart failure in these cases raise the question of an associated congenital cardiac malformation. Two cases died of heart failure, and one had a congenital malformation at autopsy. This problem was studied in the monograph of Gold et al. and others (15, 16, 17).

From the clinical standpoint we can describe 4 types:

a) Intracranial Acute Hemorrhage. After a subarachnoid hemorrhage, one patient presented with a posterior suboccipital bruit and three others had transitory neurological signs: a cerebellar syndrome in one case, and brain stem symptoms in two cases.

The intracranial hemorrhage may be a very serious emergency: the patient is comatose, decerebrate, and has repiratory failure. One case died in a few hours in spite of immediate ventricular drainage. But recovery is possible in some cases. Another patient, a housekeeper 47 years old, operated upon 8 months previously for an intracerebellar hematoma with partial resection of the angioma, had a second bleed resulting in profound coma. With conservative management she made a good recovery over three months and she is now able to work normally at home. She has had no hemorrhage for the past 8 years.

b) Long-Standing Neurological Symptoms and Signs. Headache is not a constant feature. Signs of a pyramidal tract lesion and various oculomotor palsies are the most frequent findings. In one case previously published (18), we found an alternating brain stem syndrome with a hemicerebellar affection on one side and hemianesthesia on the other with a paralysis of the IIIth and IVth cranial nerves. In two cases transient cerebellar symptoms disappeared two or three months after the subarachnoid hemorrhage.

The patient with a cerebello-pontine angle angioma had a long-standing unilateral deafness with, recently, attacks of vertigo. There was no corneal hypoesthesia nor raised intracranial pressure. X-rays were normal. A mass in the cerebello-pontine angle cistern was visible on encephalography.

Parinaud's syndrome was present in three cases, in all of whom it was transient and in two cases it occurred after subarachnoid hemorrhage. In another case, the Parinaud's syndrome appeared during pregnancy and was due to a small angioma of the quadrigeminal plate. After Caesarian section, the Parinaud's syndrome disappeared and reappeared one month later. After surgical cure of the angioma, the Parinaud's syndrome has progressively and completely disappeared.

In general, we can say that cerebellar angiomas are usually free of long-standing neurological symptoms, but that brain stem angiomas eventually lead to chronic neurological deficits.

c) Pseudotumor of the Posterior Cranial Fossa. Two cases presented with progressive cerebellar symptoms and raised intracranial pressure. In these two cases, an angioma was discovered at operation: in one case a total excision was possible, in the other a partial resection. This experience raises the question whether vertebral angiography should not be used in all patients presenting as posterior fossa tumors.

d) Hydrocephalus. This is the most common clinical presentation in infancy and related in our experience to aneurysms of the vein of Galen. This etiology must always be suspected in cases of hydrocephalus with an intracranial bruit or cardiac insufficiency or distended superficial veins of the scalp.

R a d i o l o g y

Radiological investigations must include carotid and vertebral angiography. Seldinger's technique seems the more suitable one. With pneumoencephalography there is the danger of diagnostic error and this has occurred in two of our cases. But in a case of aneurysm of the vein of Galen we could see a rounded mass in the posterior part of the ambient cistern on pneumoencephalography and this mass, which on angiography looked like a cherry, was the dilated vein of Galen.

Radiologically the differential diagnosis between these cases and hemangioblastoma of the cerebellum or the brain stem is not always very easy. The tumor cyst may be interpreted as a hematoma. Examination of the fundus rarely reveals the retinal lesion of the Von Hippel-Lindau syndrome. Polycythemia is not always present. The brain scan is positive in each case. The diagnosis can be made by analysis of the radiological pictures of the vessels. In an angioma the arterial vessels are always tortuous and dilated, and abnormal veins fill easily but in hemangioblastoma the arterial vessels are rarely dilated and if the veins do fill early, they are always in their normal position.

C o n s e r v a t i v e   T h e r a p y

7 patients have not been operated upon for different reasons or have only been explored.

2 are dead. In one case the whole illness was very rapid and lasted only a few hours. This was the first hemorrhage of a young patient, 19 years old and angiography demonstrated a small angioma of the cerebellum with hydrocephalus. The second case was a neonate presenting with congenital heart failure and obstructive hydrocephalus due to an aneurysm of the vein of Galen. He died in 4 months.

One patient is an invalid. He has a large diffuse angioma covering the whole of the base of the brain. He has never bled.

4 patients recovered and have remained well for about 5 years. All were young, between 20 and 40. Two small cerebellar angiomas had only one hemorrhage. The patient with a quadrigeminal plate angioma and an alternating brain stem syndrome, remains moderately incapacitated. She has never bled again. The last patient with an angioma of the cerebellopontine angle has never bled; he continues with attacks of vertigo.

The possibility of very long periods of health after one mild subarachnoid hemorrhage and that the neurological symptoms may not progress for many years must remain in one's mind when discussing indications for <u>surgical treatment</u>.

12 cases have been operated on with no immediate mortality.

3 patients had a suboccipital craniectomy, 9 a temporal or occipital bone flap.

In 5 cases, it was possible to extirpate completely the malformation and this was followed by a good recovery: two of these had angiomas restricted to the cerebellum (the patients were well many years later and without neurological signs); an aneurysm of the vein of Galen, resected through the right lateral ventricle (the child remains mildly retarded with rare epileptic seizures); an angioma of the quadrigeminal plate which manifested itself during pregnancy, and was resected via an occipital craniotomy after Caesarian section and a transitory Parinaud syndrome, the patient is now remaining well with only a partial homonymous hemianopsia; an angioma of the proximal posterior choroidal artery, in a girl 16 years old, resected through a temporo-occipital bone flap, and leaving a moderate hemiparesis (a hemiplegia was present before surgery).

7 cases have been submitted to partial resection or clipping of the afferent vessels. There were two mesencephalic angiomas. The first, which was very large, was in a patient who was in very poor condition when operated on and died one month after partial clipping and coagulation of the afferents. In the second patient, we could coagulate one enlarged branch which was directly fed by the mesencephalic artery through a left anterior temporal bone flap. The angioma was very thin. The patient had aphasia for a short time but is now working as an engineer. He has had no hemorrhage for three years.

One diffuse angioma extending from the cerebellum to the brain stem and cervical spinal cord was partially resected via a suboccipital craniectomy. The patient had a second hemorrhage but recovered and is still alive although with neurological deficits.

Two angiomas of the proximal posterior choroidal artery underwent partial clipping and coagulation of their blood supply through a temporo-occipital bone flap. They did well after surgery and there have been no further hemorrhages.

Two aneurysms of the vein of Galen were submitted to clipping of the afferent vessels. The first in heart failure, was operated on three times in eight months but the clips were placed too far from the lesion. He died of cardiac insufficiency. In the second case we put a clip on the afferent vessel, right under the vein of Galen, through an occipital bone flap, and there was a fairly good anatomical result. But the child remained retarded as he was before surgery. Similar observations have been made by others (19, 20).

S u m m a r y

It is possible to carry out with good results definitive surgery in some cases of cerebellar and brain stem angiomas: the aim is total resection for cerebellar angiomas, resection in a few cases of quadrigeminal plate angiomas and aneurysms of the vein of Galen, and a partial clipping in mesencephalic and posterior choroidal artery angiomas.

Results in 19 Cases
_____

No Operation: 7 Cases

    . 2 Dead
    . 4 Good Recovery
    . 1 Invalid

Operation: 12 Cases

    No Operative Mortality
    - Complete Resection: 5 Cases
    . 1 Quadrigeminal Plate
    . 1 Post. Choroidal Artery
    . 2 Cerebellum
    . 1 Aneurysm of Vein of Galen
    - 5 Good Results

    - Partial Excision or Clipping: 7 Cases

    . 2 Mesencephalic
    . 2 Post. Choroidal Artery
    . 1 Diffuse
    . 2 Aneurysm of Vein of Galen
    - 2 Died Subsequently (1 aneurysm of vein of Galen and 1 mesence-
      phalic).
    - 1 Subsequent Hemorrhage
    - 1 Bad Result
    - 3 Good Results.

_____

Angiomas of the Vertebro-Basilar System: 19 Cases
_____

Cerebellum and Vermis	: 5 Cases
Cerebello-Pontine Angle	: 1 Case
Cerebellum and Brain Stem	: 1 Case

Angiomas of the Brain Stem

1 Very Large

Quadrigeminal Plate	: 2 Cases
Mesencephalic	: 2 Cases
Posterior-Choroidal Artery:	3 Cases
(proximal)	

Aneurysm of the Vein of Galen
                            : 4 Cases

_____

R e f e r e n c e s

1. OLIVECRONA, H., RIIVES, J.: Arteriovenous aneurysms of the brain, their diagnosis and treatment. Arch. Neurol. Psychiat. (CHIC.) 59, 567-603 (1948).

2. SUTTON, D., HOARE, R. D.: Percutaneous vertebral angiography. Brit. J. Radiology. 24, 589-597 (1951).

3. LOGUE, V., MONCKTON, G.: Posterior fossa angiomas. A clinical presentation of 9 cases. Brain. 77, 252-273 (1954).

4. KRAYENBÜHL, H., YASARGIL, M. G.: Das Hirnaneurysma. 141 p. Basel: J. R. Geigy (1958).

5. LAINE, E., GALIBERT, P.: Personal communication.

6. VERBIEST, H.: Arteriovenous aneurysms of the posterior fossa. Analysis of 6 cases. Acta Neurochir. 9, 171-195 (1961).

7. BOBILLIER, P.: Les angiomes de la fosse cérébrale postérieure. A propos de 8 observations cliniques. Thèse Lyon, No 13, 46 p.(1964).

8. LAPRAS, C., TUSINI, G., THIERRY, A.: A propos de 8 observations cliniques d'angiomes de la fosse cérébrale postérieure. Congrès Soc. Neurochirurgie langue Franç. Lyon (1963).

9. LE BEAU, J., FELD, M.: Hématomes spontanés chroniques du cervelet opérés et guéris. Rev. Neurol. 79, 42-44 (1947).

10. GUILLAUME, J., SIGWALD, J., ROGE, R.: Les hématomes spontanés du cervelet. Essai de synthèse clinique. Rev. Neurol. 60, 520-521 (1948).

11. HYLAND, H. H., LEVY, D.: Spontaneous cerebellar haemorrhage. Canad. Med. Ass. J. 71, 315-323 (1954).

12. CRAWFORD, J. V., RUSSELL, D. S.: Cryptic arteriovenous and venous hamartomas of the brain. J. Neurol. Neurosurg. Psychiat. 19, 1-11 (1956).

13. MCKISSOCK, W., RICHARDSON, A., Walsh, L.: Spontaneous cerebellar hemorrhage. A study of 34 consecutive cases treated surgically. Brain 83, 1-9 (1960).

14. ODOM, G. L., TINDALL, G. T., DUKES, H. T.: Cerebellar hematoma caused by angiomatous malformations. J. Neurosurg. 6, 18, 777-782 (1961).

15. GOLD, A. P., RANSOHOFF, J., CARTER, S.: Vein of Galen malformation. Acta neurol. Scand. Suppl. 11, Vol. 40 (1964).

16. SIROT, J.: Anévrysme artério-veineux de la veine de Galien. A propos de 4 observations. Thèse Lyon, 1 vol. 74 p. (1973).

17. LAPRAS, C., BRUNAT, M.: Anévrysme de la veine de Galien. J. Med. Lyon, 617-627 (1968).

18. GIRARD, P., BONAMOUR, G., ROBERT, J., LAPRAS, C.: A propos d'une observation d'angiome à court-circuit artério-veineux de la calotte pédonculaire. Lyon Médical. 47, 817-833 (1958).

19. POOL, J. L., POTTS, D. G.: Aneurysms and arteriovenous anomalies of the brain - Diagnosis and treatment. New York - Hoeber Med. Div. - Harper and Row. I vol. 463 p. (1965).

20. MOUNT, L. A.: Arteriovenous angioma derived from the anterior inferior cerebellar artery. Its diagnosis and treatment. J. Neurosurg. 22, 612-615 (1965).

Treatment of an Angioma of the Left Cerebral Hemisphere

F. Schepelmann

The following presentation of a single case may be justified because
of its special location, its extraordinary size, and the problems
raised by the treatment of this cerebral angioma.

In this patient a slowly progressive weakness of the right limbs was
first noticed at the age of 5 years, and later hemiatrophy of the right
side of the body became apparent. Seizures began when he was 6 years
old; these were always right sided and were associated sometimes with
a speech arrest; the frequency of these seizures fluctuated from 15
a day to 6 during one year.

On examination at the age of 33 this male patient had a machinery murmur in the left temporo-parietal region of the skull. X-ray pictures
(Figs. 1, 2) showed remarkable vascularisation of the left side of the
calvarium and calcification in the left parietal region. Angiography
(Figs. 3 - 6) revealed an arteriovenous malformation of the left hemisphere in the territories of the anterior and middle cerebral arteries
occupying nearly the entire fronto-parietal region; later on an aneurysm of the basilar artery, which was not visible on the first angiogram, was found. Brain scans showed an increased emission in the posterior frontal, the anterior temporal, and the entire parietal region
on the left as well as an arteriovenous shunt. Echoencephalography recorded very large pulsating spikes on the left side. Cardiological examination disclosed a water-hammer pulse in the neck and an alteration
of the heart shape of the type seen in left ventricular stress, but the
cardiac output was in the normal range and the electrocardiogram was
normal. Neurologically there was a typical infantile hemiparesis with
hemiatrophy of the entire right side of the body, but particularly of
the right arm and the distal parts of the limbs. There was a corresponding spastic paralysis of WERNICKE-MANN type. Sensory testing found
only an alteration of position sense in the right hand. The patient
had a mild aphasia; his intellectual level was below normal. The elec-
troencephalogram showed some irregularities typical of slight general
disturbance and focal changes over the left hemisphere.

This clinical picture was demonstrated during the Annual Meeting of
the German Society for Neurosurgery in Giessen 1969. After discussion
of the therapeutic possibilities Prof. PIA performed a left hemispherectomy; at that time the patient was 35 years old. The corpus callosum
was divided paramedially on the left side and the hemisphere with the
angioma was removed including the corpus striatum and lateral parts
of the thalamus (Figs. 7, 8).

The patient was seen again 2 years after this operation. Neurologically hemianopia and hemihypaesthesia were found in addition to the hemiparesis. Moreover severe aphasia was present. Neuropsychological examination (1) revealed a serious deficit in speech particularly on the expressive side. Linguistic testing (2) also disclosed an extremely impaired performance in expression though the intention to verbalize mental concepts was well-developed. The patient was alert and entirely orientated. Based on the neuro-psychological tests (1) one could postulate that the intellectual state after the hemispherectomy was not essentially impaired in comparison with the preoperative state, but there were indications of concreteness of thought.

We must discuss whether the operative treatment of such an angioma is advisable. On the one hand this angioma occupied the largest part of that hemisphere, which we assumed to be the dominant one, and was therefore of critical importance for speech. The dominance of the left hemisphere was indicated by the attacks of speech arrest during the focal seizures as well as by the mild aphasia, which was recognized before the operation; the sodium-amytal-test did not yield useful information because of the arteriovenous shunt. On the other hand we have to take into account the fact that the non-dominant right hemisphere is also capable of some speech function and is able to take on further speech functions in case of deficits in the left hemisphere, particularly if the lesion of the left hemisphere occurred in infancy (3). We must remember that the circulatory disturbances resulting from the presence of the arteriovenous shunt would cause progressive functional impairment of the left hemisphere and consequently functional impairment of the right hemisphere (4). Moreover there was always the threat of rupture of the pathological vessels and a dangerous hemorrhage.

After the hemispherectomy dense aphasia appeared, which confirmed speech-dominance of the left hemisphere and showed that the speech-function of the right hemisphere was poor. However, the neuropsychological and linguistic examinations revealed that his intellectual state was relatively only slightly reduced after hemispherectomy.

The expressive faculties, which were lost after the operation, may be less important for the integrity of the personality than the preserved mental capacity, which probably would have become increasingly disintegrated without the operation. Taking this into consideration, we think that the treatment of such a particular cerebral angioma by hemispherectomy is advisable even if it involves the dominant hemisphere.

R e f e r e n c e s

1. BECKER, W.: Personal communication.

2. RÖSSING, H.: Personal communication.

3. POECK, K.: Die funktionelle Asymmetrie der beiden Hirnhemisphären. Dtsch. med. Wschr. 93, 2282-2287 (1968).

4. FLEISCHHACKER, H. H.: Hemispherectomy. J. Ment. Sci. 100, 66-84 (1954).

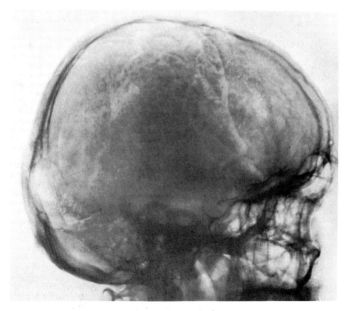

Fig. 1. Angioma of the left cerebral hemisphere.
Skull X-ray lat.

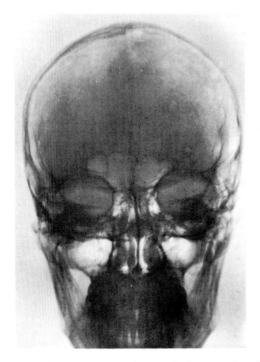

Fig. 2. Angioma of the left cerebral hemisphere.
Skull X-ray A. P.

144

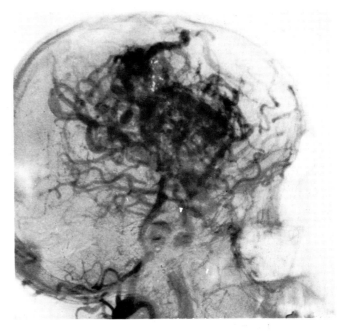

Fig. 3. Angioma of the left cerebral hemisphere.
Left brachial angiogram lat. (2.5 sec)

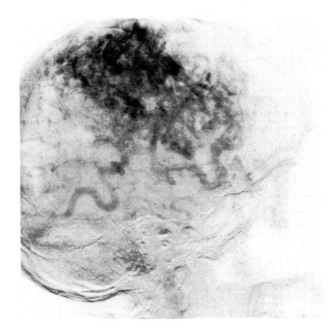

Fig. 4. Angioma of the left cerebral hemisphere.
Left brachial angiogram lat. (4.5 sec)

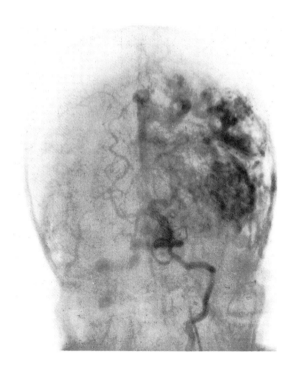

Fig. 5. Angioma of the left cerebral hemisphere
Left brachial angiogram A. P. (2.5 sec)

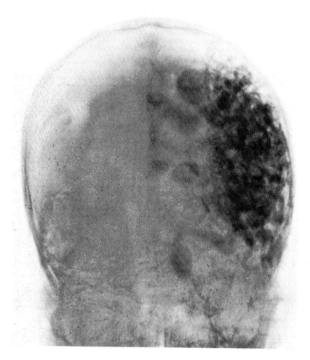

Fig. 6. Angioma of the cerebral hemisphere. Left carotid angiography
A. P. (2 sec)

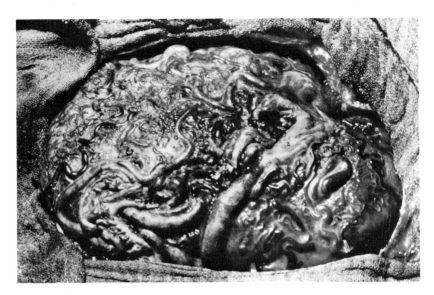

Fig. 7. Angioma of the left cerebral hemisphere
Operative view

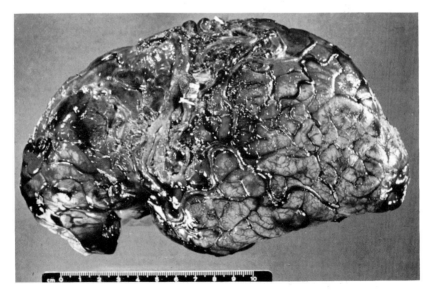

Fig. 8. Angioma of the left cerebral hemisphere
Surgical specimen after left hemispherectomy

Treatment of Cranio-Cervical Angioma. Case Report

J. ZIERSKI

The purpose of this report is to present a rare spontaneous arterio-venous malformation located mainly at the cranio-cervical junction and an unusual kyphosis, which developed after incomplete removal of the angioma.

Case Report

A 15-year-old girl (R. W., 537/72) was admitted in January 1972 with a history of 4 subarachnoid hemorrhages during the preceding 6 weeks.

On examination she was conscious and alert. There was marked neck stiffness, and she kept her head slightly rotated and flexed to the left. She had a pale angiomatous naevus on the right side of the neck, and slight pulsation over this area could be felt. There was no thrill nor audible bruit. Apart from left ankle clonus the rest of the general and neurological examination revealed no abnormalities.

Aortography, left carotid angiography, and left vertebral angiography were performed in another hospital and were considered to be normal. Right retrograde brachial angiography (Fig. 1) revealed a large congerie of vessels in the upper cervical region with a major supply from the terminal part of the right vertebral artery, muscular branches of the deep cervical artery, and possibly the external carotid circulation. The details of the malformation were difficult to define, and selective right vertebral angiography showed relatively small part of the malformation at the level of the foramen magnum.

At operation on 8.2 1972: An upper cervical laminectomy and small suboccipital craniectomy were performed. Multiple dilated vessels were ligated during the dissection of muscles. After the dura was opened, it was found that the cerebellar tonsils were herniated into the spinal canal, the veins over the exposed area were partly filled with arterial blood; on the right side of the upper cervical spinal cord, ventro-lateral, but also dorsal, there was an abnormal congerie of vessels supplied by arteries arising from the vertebral artery and running around with the first and second cervical nerve roots. Over the posterior surface of the spinal cord, the malformation merged into the system of posterior spinal arteries. Traces of old subpial bleeding were clearly seen. With the aid of the microscope the malformation was dissected and the feeders clipped. Following this, the size of angioma diminished considerably, and the remaining loops were coagulated using bipolar forceps, so that at the end of the operation it seemed that none of it was left, and the superficial cerebellar veins were again filled with venous blood.

The postoperative course was uneventful, and the patient was discharged on March 4th, 1972 in good general condition. There was minimal ataxia of gait and diminished mobility of the neck.

She was admitted for the second time 4 months later, her chief complaint being progressive increase of neck stiffness and abnormal posture of the neck. A thrill was detectable over the right side of the neck, but the remainder of the neurological examination was normal. Electromyography of the sternocleidomastoid, deep cervical, and trapezius muscles showed the pattern of tonic innervation on both sides with fibrillation potentials on the right side. Brachial angiography was repeated and showed that the malformation, though markedly diminished in size, was still present. The details of vascularisation with a supply from the dilated deep cervical artery of the costo-cervical trunk, and from the ascending cervical artery of the thyro-cervical trunk were now clearly seen (Fig. 2 a). There seemed to exist an anastomosis between the external carotid artery and the vertebral circulation. Another fact revealed was the persistence of remnants of the angioma at the terminal part of the right vertebral artery (Fig. 2 b, c).

The patient was discharged, and physiotherapeutic measures aimed at improving the posture of the neck were instituted. They were completely ineffectual, and she started to complain of intense neck pain, which was accompanied by progressive weakness of the right arm and afterwards of both legs.

Her third admission followed in January 1973. Examination revealed a spastic tetraparesis more marked on the right side. Fine movements of the fingers of the right hand were lost, the tendon reflexes on the right side were exaggerated, there was ataxia of the right arm and a positive Romberg's sign. Bilateral retrograde brachial angiography was again performed. It showed no substantial change compared with the last examination. Air and Duroliopaque myelography were performed and showed a partial block at the C 3/4 level. Between February 1972 and January 1973 considerable worsening of the kyphosis was noted, resulting finally in almost 90° forward flexion of the cervical spine (Fig. 3). Head traction with Crutchfield tongues produced a satisfactory realignment of the spine. The motor function of the right arm and the legs improved within 7 days. The patient was discharged in the beginning of April 1973, traction being changed for a cervico-thoracic brace with head support.

Two months later, while she was still wearing her brace, weakness of the right arm and a feeling of numbness reappeared. She was admitted for the fourth time in June 1973, with a severe paresis of the right arm, weakness of both legs, and bilateral patellar and ankle clonus. Marked forward flexion of the cervical spine was present again. After 10 days of traction, correct realignment was achieved, and on June, 28th an anterior fusion between C 3 and C4 was performed. Longus colli and longus capitis muscles were divided on both sides. She was discharged on September 22nd, 1973, with considerable improvement of her motor function, discrete weakness of the right hand, slight diminution of pin-prick sensation on the palmar surface of the right hand, and a trace of ataxia in the right arm. When last seen at the end of October 1973, she had no complaints and was attending her shool normally. There was no weakness and no sensory disturbance whatsoever. Her neck was practically immobile. The X-ray of the cervical spine showed good fusion between the third and fourth vertebral bodies, however, a minimal increase of forward flexion, this time centered at the C 4/5 level, was noted (Fig. 4).

D i s c u s s i o n

Spontaneous A-V malformations involving the extracranial carotid-vertebral circulation are rare. In a recent report STORRS and KING (1) mentioned 23 cases published up to 1973. Eleven of these patients were operated upon. They added 5 cases of their own out of which 4 were successfully corrected by surgery. A patient with a malformation localized within the high cervical area having a similar pattern of arterial supply (vertebral artery, subclavian artery, thyrocervical trunk, and occipital branch of the external carotid artery) as in our case was described by GREENBERG (2). In his patient surgery had to be abandoned because of a massive retrograde flow from the opposite vertebral artery. More than half of the patients reported so far have had no surgery either because the symptoms were minimal or because the lesion was considered too extensive. Spinal symptoms connected primarily with the presence of an arteriovenous malformation in the cervical area have been described, as far as we know, in only 3 patients (3, 4, 5).

The importance of selective visualization of all the major neck vessels and branches of the subclavian artery in cases of cervical arteriovenous malformations is stressed by all authors (1, 6). In our patient the extracranial part of the malformation was supplied by muscular branches of the deep cervical artery, ascending cervical artery, and the occipital branch of the external carotid artery. Branches from the vertebral artery supplied the intraspinal part of the malformation. It seems to us that only superselective angiography of the external carotid artery as described by DJINDJIAN et coll. (7) would yield some information about whether the external carotid artery participates in the supply of the intraspinal part of the angioma. This investigation is now scheduled. As far as the possibilities of complete excision of the angioma are concerned, we now feel that embolization through the feeders from the subclavian and external carotid artery combined with direct clipping of the part supplied by branches from the vertebral artery would have been the best procedure. This type of combined management of cervical A-V malformations, avoiding the otherwise considerable loss of soft tissues of the neck, has been used by STORRS and KING (1).

The kyphosis of the cervical spine, which developed in our patient after the incomplete excision of angioma, was very unusual. Signs of severe cord compression appeared as a consequence of the abnormal neck posture and disappeared completely after the proper realignment of the spine. Some degree of kyphosis is occasionally seen after extensive cervical laminectomies and is usually attributed to the division of the ligaments and disturbance of the joints. It seems that in our case the extreme kyphosis of the neck could be explained by a permanent state of increased tonus of the deep cervical musculature, and there is some evidence that this was caused by disturbed innervation due to interneuronal loss of ischaemic origin in the upper cervical segments (8).

S u m m a r y

A case of cranio-cervical angioma with an unusual kyphosis of the cervical spine is presented. Angiographic diagnosis, the problems of management, and the possible mechanism of development of the cervical kyphosis are discussed briefly.

R e f e r e n c e s

1. STORRS, D. G., KING, R. B.: Management of extracranial congenital arterio-venous malformations of the head and neck. J. Neurosurg. 38, 584-590, 1973.

2. GREENBERG, J.: Spontaneous arterio-venous malformations in the cervical area. J. Neurol. Neurosurg. Psychiat. 33, 303-309, 1970.

3. PENFIELD, W.: Discussion, in Elkin, D. C., Harris, M. H. Arteriovenous aneurysm of vertebral vessels: report of 10 cases. Ann. Surg. 124, 934-951, p. 951, 1946.

4. PYGOTT, F., HUTTON, C. F.: Angioma of the neck with intraspinal extension. Brit. J. Radiol. 37, 72-73, 1964.

5. VERBIEST, H.: Extracranial and cervical arterio-venous aneurysms of the carotid and vertebral arteries. John Hopk. Med. J. 122, 350-357, 1968.

6. LAWSON, T. L., NEWTON, T. H.: Congenital cervical arterio-venous malformations. Radiology 97, 565-570, 1970.

7. DJINDJIAN, R., COPHIGNON, J. et coll.: Embolization by superselective angiography from the femoral route in neuroradiology. Review of 60 cases. I. Technique, indications, complications. Neuroradiology, 6, 20-26, 1972.

8. SCHEPELMANN, F.: Personal communication.

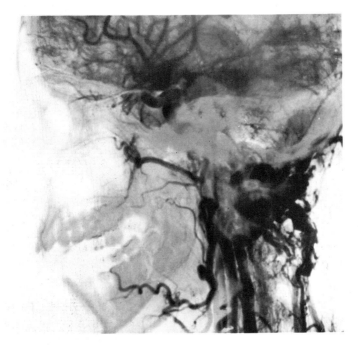

Fig. 1. R. retrograde brachial angiography. Angioma of the cranio-cervical junction

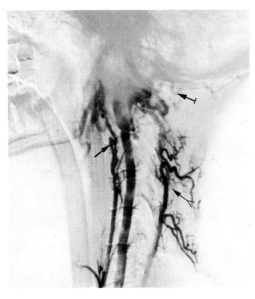

Fig. 2 a. R. retrograde brachial angiography. Lateral projection. Angioma fed by a. cervicalis ascendens (↑), occipital branch of a. carotis externa (⇡), muscular branches of the deep cervical artery (⇡)

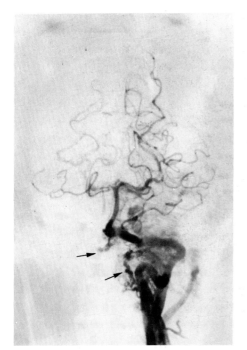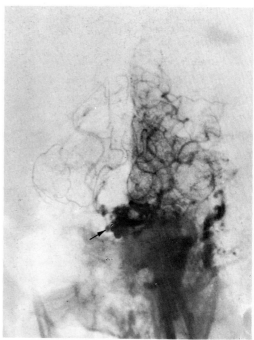

Fig. 2 b, c. b) R. retrograde brachial angiography. AP-view. Arrows point to the remnants of angioma, supplied from the R. vertebral artery. c) The same view. Later phase

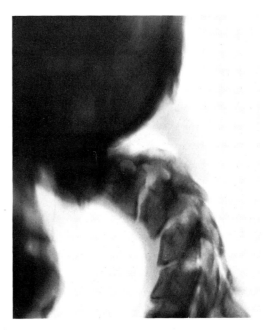

Fig. 3. Cervical spine X-ray: Tomography. Lateral view. Note the extreme kyphosis of the cervical spine at C 3/C 4 level

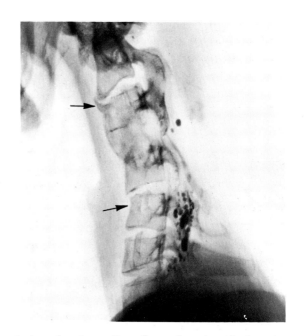

Fig. 4. Cervical spine X-ray. Lateral view. New formed osteophyte at the upper margin of C 3 (upper arrow). Slight slipping of C 4 over C 5 - one level below fusion (lower arrow)

The Acute Treatment of Cerebral Arteriovenous Angiomas Associated with Hematomas

H. W. PIA

The number of cerebro-spinal vascular anomalies has increased in the last decade due to improved knowledge of their presenting symptoms and the early use of angiography especially in cases complicated by acute hemorrhage. Our own material (Table 1) now comprises 272 a.v.-angiomas; 56 were extracerebral, 124 cerebral, and 92 spinal.

Table 1. Cerebro-spinal angiomas. The Neurosurgical University Clinic Giessen 1953-1973

Extracerebral angiomas		56
Cranial a.	30	
External carotid and ophthalmic a.	26	
Cerebral angiomas		124
Spinal angiomas		92
		272

F r e q u e n c y

Intracerebral hemorrhage is the most important complication of cerebral a.v.-angiomas. Its frequency varies between 40 and 68% in most series with an average of 52%.

	ICH	AV-Angiomas
OLIVECRONA and LADENHEIM (1957)	48	113
TÖNNIS (1957)	61	123
MCKISSOCK and HANKINSON (1957)	53	106
KUNC (1965)	48	97
AMELI (1968)	16	76
PERRET and NISHIOKA (1969)	307	545
PIA (1972)	77	124
	610	1184
	52%	

According to D. RUSSEL (27) and the review of the literature by JEL-
LINGER (6), comprising 1214 cases, hemorrhage from angiomas contrib-
utes 3-5% of spontaneous cerebral hemorrhages coming to autopsy. In his
own material of 170 cases, JELLINGER found 28 (16%) hemorrhages of angiomatous origin. These figures correlate with the clinical statistics
where they were 1145 hematomas and 213 angiomas i.e. 18.6% (JELLINGER).

In neurosurgical material the incidence is even higher and amounts to
32%, a fact which underlines their practical importance even more.

	Angiomas	ICH
KRAYENBÜHL and SIEGRFRIED (1964)	68	156
LUESSENHOP et al. (1967)	13	130
PIA (1972)	89	251
	170	537
	32%	

The so-called microangiomas (GERLACH and JENSEN (4, 5), KRAYENBÜHL and
SIEBENMANN (7)) or cryptogenic angiomas (MCCORMICK and NAFZIGER (14))
certainly contributed to these statistics, and if atypical hematomas
of uncertain origin were taken into consideration, the percentage would
be still higher.

B i o p s y   F i n d i n g s

There are few detailed reports on the different forms of intracranial
hemorrhage. Subarachnoid hemorrhage (SAH) is considered to be the most
frequent, intracerebral hematomas (ICH) are less frequent, and intraventricular hemorrhages (IVH) are only occasionally mentioned. OLIVE-
CRONA and LADENHEIM (19) found among 48 hembrrhages 39 SAH and 24 ICH.
TÖNNIS reported 40 hemorrhages without epilepsy, and 21 in combination
with seizures. Isolated or combined SAH, ICH, and IVH were found among
53 cases with hemorrhage, reported by MCKISSOCK and HANKINSON (16). In
the series of KUNC (9) there were 48 SAH and 43 ICH. KRAYENBÜHL and
YASARGIL (8) reporting 186 angiomas, found SAH in 70, ICH in 33, and
both types of bleeding in 2 cases. In the series of 37 microangiomas
reported by GERLACH (3), ICH was revealed in 31 and SAH in 19 cases.

Recurrent bleeding is quite frequent and occurs in 20-35% of the cases.
Second, third, fourth, and even more episodes are not exceptional. In
the report of PERRET and NISHIOKA (21), 81 recurrent hemorrhages are
mentioned: for the 3rd time in 13, and for the fourth time in 4 cases.
In the series of KRAYENBÜHL and YASARGIL (8) there were 53 cases of recurrent bleeding, and out of those 12 cases bled more than once. Cases
with 5 episodes of recurrent bleeding were also reported. The recurrent hemorrhage occurs after an interval of 5 years in more than 50%
of the cases, and an interval of 28 years has also been reported (TÖN-
NIS) (29).

Analysis of our material (Table 2) reveals as did our previous reports
(PIA, 24, 25) a variable picture. 77 patients had a total of 97 hemorrhages. 18 patients (19%) had previous hematomas, and almost all pa-

Table 2. Intracerebral angiomas. The type of hematoma and their localization

Localization	N		Type of Hematomas					
	Patients	Hematomas	Former H.	SAH	ICH	ICH/IVH	IVH	Sbd. H.
Frontal	5	3	—	2	—	1	—	—
Parietal	34	29	6	3	9	8	—	3
Temporal	17	10	1	—	4	4	—	1
Occipital	6	6	1	1	1	3	—	—
Hemisphere	6	2	—	2	—	—	—	—
Interhemispheric	15	12	2	2	4	4	—	—
Intratentorial	3	5	—	2	2	1	—	—
Sylvian Fissure	9	7	2	1	—	2	5	2
Basal Ganglia / Ventricle	11	15	6	—	—	3	—	—
Cerebellum	18	8	—	3	4	1	—	—
	124	97	18	17	24	27	5	6
			19%	17%	25%	28%	5%	6%

tients of this group were admitted following recurrent hemorrhage. 17
patients (17%) had subarachnoid hemorrhage, 24 patients (25%) had intracerebral hematomas, and 27 (28%) had intracerebral and intraventricular hematomas. Intraventricular hemorrhage (IVH) was present in 5
patients (5%), and subdural hematoma (Sbd.H.) in 6 (6%). Intracerebral
hematomas were the most frequent form of pathology and accounted for
53% of the total. This percentage would be even greater, if previous
hematomas, which were diagnosed only on clinical grounds, were included.

Of 30 patients with intracerebral hematomas 8 had blood-stained CSF,
and in 22 cases the CSF was normal. Blood-stained CSF (SAH) was found
in 30 cases where intraventricular hemorrhage had occurred either in
isolation or in combination with other types. Also the 6 patients with
subdural hematomas had blood-stained CSF. There were 20 ventricular
hemorrhages. In 9 cases the ventricle of which the wall was ruptured
was blocked by prolapsed choroid plexus. 9 patients had hematomas of
the ipsilateral ventricle or of parts of the lateral ventricle (partial tamponade of the ventricle). In 2 cases the foramen of Monroe
was blocked.

These clinical data seem to suggest that in cases of arteriovenous
angiomas blood-stained CSF indicates that it is more likely that an
intracerebral hematoma has ruptured into the ventricle than that the
blood has entered the cerebral subarachnoid space (SAH). The frequency
of isolated ventricular bleeding is low due to the rare occurrence of
intraventricular angiomas in general.

A g e   a n d   S e x   D i s t r i b u t i o n

Table 3. Intracerebral angiomas. Associated with hematomas - age and
sex

| Age | N | Sex | | N. of Cases | | N |
				No Hematomas	Hematomas	Hematomas
10	16	8	8	6	10	11
20	17	10	7	5	12	17
30	23	17	6	10	13	18
40	36	23	13	16	20	23
50	18	11	7	6	12	15
60	9	7	2	2	7	10
>60	5	3	2	2	3	3
	124	79	45	47	77	97
		64%	36%	38%	62%	

The age distribution (Fig. 1 and Table 3) shows that almost three quar-
ters of the hemorrhages occur within the first 4 decades of life. In
our own material there is a peak in the 4th decade, the frequency of
hemorrhage in each decade until then being no higher than in older age
groups. The data from the cooperative study showed that 82% of hemorrhages occurred in younger age groups with the highest percentage i.e.

85% in the second decade of life. In older age groups the frequency drops to 61%. In both sets of statistics the absolute peak falls in the fourth decade of life, though in the series of TÖNNIS (29) in the second and third decade of life. The relatively high incidence of hemorrhage from angiomas in the older age groups is noteworthy, however, and this may be of importance in the differential diagnosis. There were no significant differences with regard to the sex distribution.

As far as the type of hemorrhage is concerned (Table 4), intraventricular hemorrhage from intraventricular angiomas occurred exclusively before the age of 40, and intracerebral and combined intracerebral intraventricular hematomas also fell mainly within the same age limit. Recurrent bleeding and subarachnoidal bleeding was seen relatively frequently in older patients.

Table 4. Intracerebral angiomas. Type of hematomas and age

Age	N Hematomas	Type of Hematomas Former H.	SAH	ICH	ICH IVH	IVH	Sbd. H.
10	11	–	1	3	5	1	1
20	17	5	2	4	5	1	–
30	18	1	4	8	2	1	2
40	23	3	3	6	8	2	1
50	15	7	3	1	4	–	–
60	10	2	3	1	2	–	2
>60	3	–	1	1	1	–	–
	97	18	17	24	27	5	6
		19%	17%	25%	28%	5%	6%

S i t e   a n d   S i z e   o f   A n g i o m a s

The site of the angioma (Fig. 2) has considerable bearing on the occurrence of bleeding. Hemorrhage occurs most frequently from angiomas situated medially, in the interhemispheric sulcus, intratentorially, in the Sylvian fissure, in the basal ganglia, or in the ventricles rather than from angiomas located peripherally in the cerebral hemispheres. Hemorrhage is least frequent from huge angiomas of the cerebral hemispheres and from angiomas of the cerebellum. Recurrent bleeding is most frequent in angiomas of the parietal region and angiomas located centrally in the ventricles and basal ganglia (Table 5). Subarachnoid bleeding and subdural hematomas are most frequent with angiomas located near the cortex. Hemorrhage into the white matter occurs predominantly in the parietal, temporal, and occipital regions. Rupture of the hematoma into the ventricle is almost invariable in cases of massive hemorrhage from deep-seated angiomas, but is an exception in arteriovenous malformations of the cerebellum (Table 2).

There is a relationship between frequency of hemorrhage and the size of the angioma. In agreement with PATERSON and MCKISSOCK (20) among others, and the reports on the microangiomas, we found (Table 6) that

small and very small angiomas up to the size of a cherry show a specific tendency to bleed, whereas large and very large angiomas show much
less tendeny to rupture, and compared with the small malformations,
which usually produce recurrent hemorrhage, the course when they do
rupture is usually not dangerous.

Table 5. Location of cerebral angiomas and hematomas

| Localization | N | N. of cases | | N |
		No Hematoma	Hematomas	Hematomas
Frontal	5	2	3	3
Parietal	34	10	24	29
Temporal	17	8	9	10
Occipital	6	1	5	6
Hemisphere	6	5	1	2
Interhemispheric	15	4	11	12
Intratentorial	3	–	3	5
Sylvian Fissure	9	4	5	7
Basal Ganglia / Ventricle	11	2	9	15
Cerebellum	18	11	7	8
Total	124	47	77	97

Table 6. Size of angiomas and frequency of hematomas

| | N | Size | | | | |
		Large	Walnut	Cherry	Bean	Micro
No Hematoma	47	28	10	7	1	1
Former Hematomas	16	9	5	–	2	–
Acute Hematomas	61	7	8	26	14	6

Symptomatology and Course

The type and progress of a hemorrhage from an angioma are reflected
in the clinical and CSF findings. Thus an acute apoplectic onset with
severe neurological deficit, such as hemiplegia, aphasia, hemianopia
etc., with disturbances of consciousness and coma, with signs of acute
elevation of the intracranial pressure and mesencephalic or bulbar
herniation, and/or secondary deterioration with loss of central vege-
tative and metabolic control suggest an intracerebral hematoma. In
these cases blood-stained CSF would suggest probable rupture into the
ventricle. On the other hand, it is impossible to exclude an intracranial hemorrhage because the acute neurological deficits are transient
or slight or because severe focal deficits are unaccompanied by coma
or because there is a subacute course reminiscent of a tumor. Headache
as well as neck stiffness and other signs of meningeal irritation may
be lacking even in patients with blood-stained CSF.

It is generally assumed that the course and prognosis of this type of hemorrhage is relatively benign and that even large hematomas which do not produce severe deficits can show spontaneous recovery. In our experience, one of the reasons for this is the frequency of their rupture into the ventricle, which facilitates the absorption of the hematoma. Massive bleeding into the ventricular system with lethal total tamponade of the plexus is prevented by the chorioidal plexus blocking the rupture of the Foramen of Monro. We have presented evidence of such protective function of the plexus in earlier reports (PIA, 24, 25).

Out of the 247 cases of hemorrhage collected in the cooperative study (PERRET and NISHIOKA)(21), 90 patients had a hemiparesis, 28 hemiplegia, 6 facial weakness, 2 speech troubles, and 4 hemianopia, i.e. 53% of the patients had neurological deficits as a result of the first bleed. Out of 22 of NORLEN'S (18) patients one was seen in the acute stage, 3 in the subacute, and 18 during a symptom-free interval. Out of 16 patients reported by AMELI (1), 11 had a progressive history over 2 weeks to 3 months of increasing intracranial pressure and papilledema. Only in 5 cases was the onset of symptoms acute, followed by spontaneous improvement.

Our own material comprises 57 acute hematomas (21 ICH, 29 ICH and IVH, 4 certain and 3 possible IVH).

An extremely acute course was observed in 13 patients, 11 of whom had a history of less than 24 hours, and 2 of two days duration. With the exception of a single case, all patients were in coma, and 9 of them showed signs of mesencephalic, and one patient additionally signs of bulbar compression with respiratory paralysis and severe neurological deficits. In 10 cases the hematoma was localized to the parietal region, but in the remaining cases it was situated in the interhemispheric fissure and the brain stem, or in the cerebellum. 10 patients had ICH and IVH, 4 of them with tamponade of the ventricle, and 2 with prolapse of the plexus; 2 patients had ICH, one of them combined with SAH and Sbd. H.; and finally one patient had an IVH. Secondary deterioration occurred in 3 patients, 2 developing slight symptoms a few days after the occurrence of the hemorrhage.

An acute course with a history of about one week was observed in 7 patients. Disturbances of consciousness were seen in 4 of them, and signs of mesencephalic compression were found in 2. One patient deteriorated secondarily after an acute onset. In this group of patients, the hematoma was found in the parietal and occipital lobe 5 times, in the interhemispheric fissure in one patient and in the basal ganglia in another. With the exception of a single case, all the other patients had ICH with IVH. 3 patients had tamponade of the ventricle, and in 2 cases prolapse of the plexus was revealed.

A subacute course with a history of some 2 weeks was seen in 13 patients. 6 of them were in coma, 2 had disturbances of consciousness, 2 had signs of brain-stem compression, and one showed progressive deterioration. In the remaining patients there was a tendency to spontaneous improvement following an acute onset. In 6 cases the hematomas were located in the frontal or parietal lobes, in 3 cases in the basal ganglia or ventricles, in 2 cases in the Sylvian fissure, in one case in the interhemispheric fissure, and in one case infratentorially. 4 patients had an ICH, the remaining ones ICH and IVH, 3 of them with ventricle tamponade, and 2 with prolapse of the plexus.

A subacute or chronic course with a history of 2 weeks to 3 months was observed in 24 patients. With the exception of 5 patients, all had an

acute onset with coma in 10 cases, and disturbances of consciousness
in 4 followed by spontaneous improvement of the cerebral symptoms. 5
patients had focal neurological deficits as the acute initial symptoms.
The hemorrhage was localized in 9 cases to the cerebral hemisphere,
mainly in the temporal lobe, in 2 cases at the tentorial hiatus, in 4
cases in the ventricle and basal ganglia, and in one case in the Sylvian fissure. The remaining hematomas were localized with one exception in the cerebellum, and in 5 cases a large part of the hematoma
was found in the interhemispheric fissure. 14 patients had an ICH, one
ICH and IVH, 3 an IVH, one ventricular tamponade, and 2 prolapse of
the chorioidal plexus.

It can be said that intracerebral hematomas with or without rupture
into the ventricle and ventricular bleeding have, with few exceptions,
an acute onset, and in a quarter of the cases an extremely acute course,
in 10% an acute course, in another quarter a subacute course, and in
40% of cases a subacute or chronic course. Secondary deterioration, as
seen in 6 patients, and a course reminiscent of a tumor observed in 5
patients, were rare. With the exception of the extremely acute and of
the majority of the acute forms, improvement in the general cerebral
symptoms and in the focal neurological deficits in many is the rule.
Focal neurological signs and the displacement of vessels seen on angiography constituted a further indication for operation in the latter
group of patients. Intracerebral hematomas of parietal localization
with rupture into the ventricle have a tendency towards an extremely
acute course. Hemorrhage from angiomas in the basal ganglia and ventricles or in the interhemispheric fissure and the cerebellum, and
particularly when it is accompanied by intracerebral hematoma formation and intraventricular hemorrhage, has for the most part a subacute
or mild course.

It is superfluous to discuss here the importance of angiography in the
diagnosis of a hematoma and in establishing its origin. From our experience immediate angiography is essential not only in patients of
the younger age groups with an extremely acute course to their illness,
but also in the other cases with an apoplectic onset followed by a progressive and then regressive course. Older patients should undergo angiography after stabilization of the signs of central dysregulation.
This concept of management has influenced and underlain our own active
approach.

It is of course not difficult to recognize the larger hematomas. Focal
slowing of the cerebral circulation and evidence of isolated vessel
displacement will give almost certain indication about the site of the
smaller hematomas. Ventricular hemorrhages are difficult to verify;
displacement and stretching of the central arteries, particularly of
the insular group, and of the central veins may indicate tamponade of
the ventricle, in such cases blood-stained CSF will be most helpful
in suggesting that bleeding has taken place into the ventricle.

I n d i c a t i o n s   f o r   S u r g e r y

Intracerebral hemorrhage and particularly recurrent hemorrhage is regarded by all authors as an indication for operation in order to protect the patient from further bleeding. As far as special problems
are concerned, for instance the timing of operation, the type of procedure, and the contraindications to surgery, these are only seldom
discussed.

In view of the death of a patient operated upon in coma during the acute phase, and satisfactory results obtained in 3 patients operated upon during the subacute stage and 18 patients operated upon during the symptom-free interval, NORLEN (18) advises against early operation. KRAYENBÜHL and YASARGIL (8) are of the same opinion. TÖNNIS (29) saw no indications for surgery in 5 cases in coma. MCKISSOCK and HANKINSON (16) consider that surgery is particularly indicated for small angiomas with one or more hemorrhages and that it should be done early in acute hemorrhage. FRENCH and CHOU (21) in their review point out that the presence of a hematoma should be regarded as an indication for operation for functional and life-saving reasons. Similarly other authors have reported that total extirpation of the angioma is easier in the presence of a hematoma separating it from the cerebral tissue.

In the last 7 years we and our colleagues from the neurological and medical centre have tried to improve the prognosis of acute disturbances of the cerebral circulation through the earliest possible diagnosis, early conservative and operative treatment and continuous intensive care, supervision and therapy. In another place (PIA 24, 25) we discussed the importance of treatment in the acute phase in patients with hemorrhage caused by angiomas. Detailed analysis has, however, not yet been published.

Therapeutic Measures

With few exceptions the evacuation of intracerebral and intraventricular clots and total extirpation of the angioma at the same time proved to be possible and relatively simple. Due to the damage of the cerebral tissues surrounding the angioma, the latter was mostly isolated, was lying free and could be extirpated in the usual manner. The approach can be limited and the cerebral tissue protected by the use of the operation microscope in cases with more deeply situated angiomas and hematomas. The acute hematoma can be fairly easily removed by washing it out under slight pressure (Fig. 3, 4). In such a way an additional damage to the already compressed and hyperaemic surrounding brain tissue can be almost completely avoided. The patient is thus protected from secondary damage caused by raised intracranial pressure and there is a better chances for the improvement of functional deficits than in an operation carried out at a later stage.

Prognosis

According to the earlier reports, the prognosis for operative treatment of hemorrhages from angiomas is relatively good. In MCKISSOCK's (17) series of 68 patients with angiomas totally extirpated 59 patients had an isolated or combined SAH, ICH, and IVH, and 53 of the recovered. In the statistics of PERRET and NISHIOKA (21) comprising 148 operated cases, 18 patients (12%) died, 10 of them had paraventricular angiomas, 3 midline malformations, and 5 patients had huge hemispheric angiomas. In 119 cases total extirpation of the angioma was performed. Out of this number 13 patients (11%) died. Of 7 patients who had a carotid ligation, one died, of 12 patients, who had only evacuation of the hematoma three died, and of 10 patients who had ligation of the proximal feeding vessels one died. The follow-up of surviving patients showed that 53 were in good general condition, whereas 16 patients had severe deficits.

163

The overall mortality due to the intracerebral hemorrhage leading to admission to hospital was 10% (29 cases out of 281). Of 103 patients who were treated conservatively 13% died (13 patients); 44% had no or slight neurological deficits, 19% were moderately, and 10% severely disabled.

On the basis of our own material we have tried to analyse the importance on the prognosis of the timing of the operation, of the clinical symptoms, and of the location and size of the angioma and hematoma.

Of 57 cases of hematoma 53 were operated upon (Table 7). 8 patients (i.e. 15%) died. In the group of 16 patients with signs of mesencephalic herniation and decerebration there were 7 deaths, and in the group of 29 patients who were in coma 6 died. Of 12 patients with a hyper-acute course 6 died. In the group of patients with signs of decerebration 4 died in spite of immediate evacuation of the hematoma through burr holes. 2 patients died later, one after a few days, due to midbrain hemorrhage, and the other surviving for half a year in a decorticate condition. The remaining 6 patients were saved by immediate surgery.

One of them was a 20-year-old male (A. Sch. 944/64) with a cherry-sized pariet-occipital angioma, a huge intracerebral hematoma and tamponade of the lateral ventricle, who was operated upon a few hours after the acute onset of the hemorrhage which was followed by rapid deterioration. His general condition is now entirely satisfactory, and he has only a slight hemiparesis (Fig. 5).

The second case was a 7-year-old girl (C. K. 614/66) with a cherry-sized cerebellar angioma, and an intracerebellar hematoma which had ruptured into the fourth ventricle. She had a history of an acute pain in the head and neck 24 hours prior to admission followed shortly afterwards by coma, disturbances of posture, and bilateral ankle clonus. On admission, she was comatose, without neck stiffness, but the reflexes in the extremities were absent though she had bilateral plantar extensor responses. Echoencephalography showed the third ventricle to be 1 cm wide. Shortly after admission the pupils became dilated without reaction to light. She became decerebrate, and respiration ceased. Immediate angiography was carried out followed by the evacuation of a 40 cc hematoma from the left cerebellar hemisphere and removal of blood clots from the fourth ventricle. The angioma was totally extirpated. The postoperative course was uneventful, and the girl at present has no deficits (Fig. 6).

A further example is that of a 57-year-old male (L. R. 987/ 76) with a small temporal angioma, a subdural hematoma, an ICH of 40 cc, a ventricular hemorrhage, and prolapse of the plexus. The patient presented the symptoms of midbrain compression. In the acute phase the hematomas were removed. In the second stage, 3 months later, the angioma was totally extirpated. His postoperative course was uneventful, and the patient has continued to work as a priest for the past 5 years.

Of the remaining 41 patients with acute and subacute course following the hemorrhage we lost 2, i.e. 5%.

The first case was a 31-year-old patient (N. K. 447/64) with a cherry-sized tentorial angioma of the posterior cerebral and chorioidal arteries, hemorrhage into the temporal lobe, and tamponade of the ventricles. He was operated upon 10 days after the onset of the hemorrhage whilst in coma with unreactive pupils and signs of midbrain compres-

Table 7. Cerebral angiomas and acute hematomas – Operative prognosis

Time of Operation	N	Brain Stem Symptoms	Consciousness			Operation		Sur-vived	Dead
			Coma	Semi-coma	Con-scious	P	Total Extirpat.		
24 hours	10	7	9	–	1	3	7	5	5
2 days	2	2	2	–	–	1	1	1	1
1 week	6	2	2	3	1	–	6	6	–
2 weeks	12	2	6	1	5	2	10	11	1
2 weeks	23	3	10	2	11	2	21	22	1
	53	16	29	6	18	8	45	45	8
		(7)	(6)	(1)	(1)	(4)	(4)	85%	15%

sion. He died two months after operation while in a relatively satisfactory state due to pulmonary complications.

The second case was a 55-year-old male (H. L. 623/66) with an angioma
in the same location, and with a hematoma in the cerebral peduncle.
He did not lose consciousness. He was operated upon three wekks after
the hemorrhage, and died two weeks after the operation. The autopsy
revealed old and recent infarction of basal ganglia, midbrain, and
pons.

39 patients survived, and with a few exceptions, are at present in
satisfactory or good general condition, and continue to work.

Particularly impressive was the reversebility or marked improvement of
severe deficits even in cases with large hematomas. Of 8 patients with
one frontal, one temporal, and 6 parietal hematomas of volume between
100 and 250 cc, one patient has died. The remainder with one exception
regained full working capacity. 2 of them occupy university positions,
one took his degree 2 years after the operation. 2 patients recovered
without residual signs, 4 remained with a moderate or slight hemiparesis, and one patient with a hematoma of 250 cc (Figs. 7, 8) has a
severe hemiparesis. It is worthwhile mentioning that hemiplegia or
aphasia, and hemianopia of sudden onset occurred in 2 cases without
any disturbance of consciousness, and in one case with only slight
drowsiness. Three of the above mentioned 8 patients were operated upon
within 24 hours, four within one week, and one 6 weeks after the hemorrhage.

Table 8. Location of hematomas and prognosis

	2 Days		2 Weeks		>2 Weeks	
	N	Dead	N	Dead	N	Dead
Frontal Parietal	10	6	8	-	3	-
Temporal Occipital	1	-	3	-	5	-
Inter-Hemispheric	-	-	2	-	5	-
Intra-Tentorial	-	-	1	1	2	1
Sylvian Fissure Basal Ganglia	-	-	4	-	4	-
Cerebellum	1	-	-	-	4	-

The localization of the angioma and hematoma (Table 8) is important
insofar as the fatalities occurred in the acute stage only in cases
where the clot was situated in the frontal and parietal lobes and in
one case within the tentorium but with mild clinical course. In both
these groups the mortality rate of 6 out of 27, and 2 out of 3 patients
respectively, is quite high. Death was caused by direct and indirect
damage to the brain stem, particularly the midbrain.

Extensive lesions of the basal ganglia and thalamus seemed to be tolerated quite well, and were connected with relatively minor neurological deficits.

One of our patients was a 45-year-old male (H. W. 5082/59)with a large
angioma within the temporal lobe and basal ganglia. He had 2 hemorrhages 16 and 10 years prior to admission to our clinic, and each time
a hemiparesis and hemianopia with blood-stained CSF were observed.
Ligation of the carotid artery performed after the first hemorrhage
increased the hemiparesis. His last admission followed the hemorrhage
10 days before, which destroyed large parts of the temporal lobe, internal capsule, and basal ganglia with penetration of the ventricle.
Evacuation of the hematoma and total extirpation of the angioma produced chronic pain of thalamic type in the paralysed extremities. He
has been followed up for a further 14 years and his present condition
is satisfactory with a residual hemiparesis and incomplete hemianopia.

Another patient (B. S. 389/73) was a 44-year-old female who had an
angioma of the left Sylvian fissure and intracranial bleeding 30 years
ago accompanied by coma and hemiplegia from which she recovered. Since
that time she has had occasional focal seizures with transient paresis of the hand. The present hemorrhage destroyed parts of the insula,
external and internal capsules, and basal ganglia, and produced tamponade of the lateral ventricle. The onset was acute with coma, hemiplegia, decerebration, and signs of midbrain compression. During the
next days she made a slight spontaneous recovery and was operated on
ten days after the hemorrhage. Her mental condition is at present absolutely normal, her general condition is good, but she still has a
marked hemiparesis.

The influence of the type of the hematoma (Table 9) is of little significance and correlates well with the relatively benign course of
ventricular bleeding.

The mortality rates in ICH and ICH combined with IVH are similar. 2
patients of the latter group, in whom unfortunately no autopsy was
performed, died probably because of complete tamponade of the ventricles. Among 4 cases of ventricular hematoma there was no mortality.

An interesting observation was made in a 18-year-old female (G. C.
424/69) with a parietal cherry-sized round angioma, and hematoma of
100 cc which ruptured into the ventricle. The onset of the illness
was acute with coma lasting for 2 days, clouding of consciousness for
a further week, and hemiplegia. She was admitted 6 weeks after the
hemorrhage. During the operation an encapsuled, partially resorbed
hematoma with a 15 mm wide rupture was found to be closed by the plexus. Histological examination of this tissue showed the formation of
small cysts, thrombosis of dilated stromal vessels, and degenerative
changes caused by compression which confirmed the efficacy of the
block and the protective function of the chorioidal plexus.

The age of patient does not seem to have any influence on the mortality.
Of 5 patients aged over 55 years one has died. The remaining patients,
aged 55, 57, 62, and 65 survived in good condition.

The removal of the hematoma and total extirpation of the angioma at
one operation appears to be the optimal method and at the same time
the least dangerous.

Table 9. Type of intracerebral hematoma and operative prognosis

Time of operation	N	Intracerebral Hematom.		Intracerebral and		Ventricular H.	
		N	†	N	†	N	†
24 hours	10	2	2	8	3	-	-
2 days	2	-	-	2	1	-	-
1 week	6	1	-	5	-	-	-
2 weeks	12	4	-	7	1	1	-
>2 weeks	23	14	1	6	-	3	-
	53	21	3	28	5	4	-
			14,5%		18%		

Evacuation of the hematoma by needling and aspiration is by comparison
with the previous method less efffective, but can be of advantage in
certain cases.

In 4 patients with an extremely acute course operation could not prevent a fatal outcome because of irreversible damage to the brain stem.
In 3 patients with deep-seated paraventricular angiomas the evacuation
of the hematoma saved their lives.

Another patient, a 65-year-old male (K. W. 717/63) with an angioma of
the Sylvian fissure and temporal hematoma, which ruptured into the
temporal horn was admitted 6 weeks after the acute onset of drowsiness,
hemiplegia, and hemianopia. Lumbar puncture revealed blood-stained CSF.
Aspiration of the hematoma resulted in an almost complete neurological
recovery though there remained some impairment of mental efficiency.

Special anaesthetic methods are not necessary for the management of
intracerebral hemorrhage due to angiomas. For many years we used hypo-
thermia between 30 and 28° C, temporary clamping of carotids, and
artificial arterial hypotension, but the analysis showed that these
measures had no particular advantage. We operate upon our patients
under standard Halothane anaesthesia, and occasionally use additional
hypotensive measures. We consider the best pre- and postoperative supervision and treatment in an Intensive-Care-Unit to be most important.

C o n c l u s i o n s

Our observations confirm the necessity for active management of arteriovenous malformations complicated by hematomas. An extremely acute
course with rapid increase of intracranial pressure, and signs of midbrain or medullary compression was present in 25% of our patients.
Even so, it was possible to save half of them. In the remaining patients with an acute or subacute course, the evacuation of the hematoma and total extirpation of the angioma in a one stage procedure
was associated with the least possible risk. Taking into consideration
the fact that the natural course of such hematomas is frequently
straightforward and that the signs show a continuous regression, the
improvement in the most severe deficits which follows surgery, the
elimination of the dangers of secondary damage caused by raised pressure, and the elimination of recurrent hemorrhage, are all in favour
of early operation. Since small and tiny angiomas constitute the majority of cases and have a particular tendency to bleed, early operation is even more strongly indicated. The destruction of the surrounding tissue by the hematoma is not a limiting factor in cases of
angiomas in functionally important regions and in deep-lying structures, but on the contrary, it decreases the risk of the operation.
The extirpation of the malformation is easier due to the isolation
of the angioma from the surrounding tissues by the blood-clot. Additional damage is an exceptional occurrence provided the correct operative technique is followed and the operation microscope is used. Needling and aspiration of the hematoma is still of value in few selected cases. As opposed to the view which is sometimes expressed, bleeding from an angioma occurs mostly into the brain tissue or into the
ventricle, and rarely into the subarachnoid space. The localizing
signs of a circumscribed space occupying lesion can always be found,

but the signs of a general increase of intracranial pressure may be absent. However, if the latter are present, they do not militate against operation. Decompression achieved by evacuation of the hematoma and total extirpation of the angioma, performed in a one-stage procedure combines the curative and prophylactic side of management.

It seems to me that we have shown that the hyper-acute and acute stages after bleeding from an angioma should not be regarded as contraindications to surgery, but, on the contrary, as indication for early operation. In long-standing cases where there is a tendency to spontaneous improvement, the indication for decompressive procedure recedes into the background as compared with the resection of the angioma in order to prevent further hemorrhage. As far as the so-called inoperable angiomas are concerned, it seems to me that to-day we cannot accept that those which are most dangerous from the vital and functional point of view are inoperable though there are complications in this group of arteriovenous malformations.

S u m m a r y

The report deals with 77 cases of intracerebral hemorrhage, which occurred in 124 patients with cerebral arteriovenous malformations. These constitute part of a series of 272 cerebro-spinal angiomas. The problem of the management of the acute stage following hemorrhage from an angioma is discussed. The incidence of such hemorrhage increased from 52 to 62% due to better and earlier diagnosis. In an autopsy survey of spontaneous intracerebral hematoma, hemorrhage from arteriovenous malformation was found in 5%, whereas in clinical statistics it occurred in 18%, and in statistics from neurosurgical centres in 32%. In opposition to the data so far published, intracerebral hematomas alone and in combination with ventricular hematomas constituted 25% and 28% of all forms of intracerebral hemorrhage respectively. Thus they represented the most frequent form of intracranial bleeding i.e. 53%. Subarachnoidal hemorrhage occurred in 19%, subdural hematomas in 6%, and intraventricular hemorrhage by itself in 5%. Recurrent bleeding occurred in 30% of the cases. Blood-stained CSF is primarily an indication of hemorrhage into the ventricular system.

Three-quarters of the hemorrhage from angiomas occur within the first four decades of life with a peak in the fourth decade. The relatively high frequency of hemorrhages in the older age groups emphasizes the importance of differential diagnosis. Small and tiny angiomas and angiomas of the midline (in the interhemispheric fissure, the ventricle, the basal ganglia, the Sylvian fissure, and the tentorial hiatus) have a higher tendency to bleed than huge hemispheric angiomas and angiomas of the cerebellum.

The clinical picture is characterized by an apoplectic onset and severe neurological deficit. An extremely acute clinical course of a few hours duration was seen in 25% of cases. 10% of cases had an acute course lasting approximately one week and showed an acute increase of intracranial pressure. 25% of cases had a subacute course lasting up to 2 weeks, and 40% a chronic course with a history lasting from 2 weeks to 3 months. In the latter groups an acute onset was followed by a tendency to continuous improvement of the cerebral symptoms combined with some improvement of the focal neurological signs. A pseudotumoral course is exceptional. Cerebral angiography reveals the presence of the angioma and local, as well as general, displacement of the intra-cranial vessels. Rupture of the hematoma into the ventricle is ascertained by lumbar puncture, which shows a blood-stained CSF.

Our active approach comprising early diagnosis and early operation is supported by the analysis of the results of treatment. Of 12 patients with an extremely acute course, 6 have died, 4 with irreversible brain stem damage and after aspiration of the hematoma. 6 patients were saved. Of the remaining 41 patients, 2 died, one due to pulmonary complications and another due to midbrain infarction. Angiomas located in the parietal lobe and in the tentorial hiatus have a particularly high mortality (6 deaths out of 27 cases, and 2 deaths out of 3 cases, respectively). The simultaneous presence of hemorrhage confined to the ventricle or of ventricular tamponade does not constitute an additional risk. In many cases the closure of the site of rupture by the prolapse of the chorioidal plexus facilitates the resorption of the hematoma and explains the relatively mild clinical course. The age of the patient and the size of the angioma have little significance for the mortality. Of 8 patients with huge hematomas of 100 to 250 cc, one died. Improvement of the neurological function, and cure in the majority of cases, underlines the importance of early operation to prevent secondary damage produced by increased intracranial pressure. Evacuation of the hematoma and total extirpation of the angioma (carried out in 45 out of 53 cases) protect the patients from recurrent bleeding and circulatory damage. Local damage to the brain tissue caused by hematomas facilitates the resection of the angioma, particularly of the deep-lying ones. The operative procedure is facilitated by microsurgical techniques. Evacuation of the hematoma by needling and aspiration is indicated only in a few cases.

Bleeding from an angioma is a straightforward indication for early surgery, which lessens the mortality in the extremely acute cases and generally improves morbidity. Operative mortality is low. Only in exceptional cases can the patient who has bled from an angioma be considered inoperable.

References

1. AMELI, N. O.: Brain angiomata and intracerebral hematoma. In Progr. Brain Research 30, 427-431. Amsterdam-London-New York: Elsevier 1968.

2. FRENCH, L. A., CHOU, S. N.: Conventional Methods of Treating Intra-cranial Arteriovenous Malformations. Progr. Neurosurg. 3, 275-361 (1969). Basel-New York: S. Karger.

3. GERLACH, J.: Intracerebral Hemorrhage. Caused by Microangiomas. Progr. neurol. Surg. 5, 363-396 (1969).

4. GERLACH, J., JENSEN, H. P.: Mikroangiome des Gehirns. Arch. klin. Chir. 293, 481-493 (1960).

5. GERLACH, J., JENSEN, H. P.: Die intracerebralen Haematome bei Mikroangiomen. Acta Neurochir., Suppl. 7, 367-373 (1961).

6. JELLINGER, K.: Zur Ätiologie und Pathogenese der spontanen intra-zerebralen Blutung. Therapiewoche 22, 1440-1450 (1972).

7. KRAYENBÜHL, H., SIEBENMANN, R.: Small vascular malformations as a cause of primary intracerebral hemorrhage. J. Neurosurg. 22, 1-20 (1965).

8. KRAYENBÜHL, H., YASARGIL, M. G.: Klinik der Gefäßmißbildungen und Gefäßfisteln. In H. Gänshirt: Der Hirnkreislauf, S. 465-511. Stuttgart: Thieme 1972.

9. KUNC, Z.: Possibility of surgery in arteriovenous malformations in the anatomically important and dangerous regions of the brain. J. Neurol. Neurosurg. Psychiat. 28, 183 (1965).

10. LAINE, E., DELANDSHEER, GALIBERT, P., et al.: Hématomes intracérébraux spontanés profonds (en particulier du noyau caudé) en rapport avec des malformations angiomateuses (télangiactasis et cavernomes). Etude angiographique et déduction thérapeutique. Neurochir. 2, 340-355 (1956).

11. LAZORTHES, G.: Les hémorrhagies intracraniennes: Traumatiques, spontanées et du premier âge. 256 pp. Paris: Masson & Cie. 1952.

12. LAZORTHES, G.: L'hémorrhagie cérébrale. Vue par le Neurochirurgien. Paris: Masson & Cie. 1956.

13. LAZORTHES, G.: Surgery of cerebral hemorrhage. Report on the results of 52 surgically treated cases. J. Neurosurg. 16, 355-364 (1959).

14. MCCORMICK, W. F., NAFZINGER, J. D.: "Cryptic" vascular malformations of the central nervous system. J. Neurosurg. 24, 865-875 (1966).

15. MCKISSOCK, W., RICHARDSON, A., WALSH, L.: Spontaneous cerebellar haemorrhage. A study of 34 consecutive cases treated surgically. Brain 83, 1-9 (1960).

16. MCKISSOCK, W., HANKINSON, J.: The surgical treatment of the supratentorial angiomas. Rapports et discussions. 1er Congrès International de Neurochirurgie, Bruxelles 1957.

17. MCKISSOCK, W., RICHARDSON, A., TAYLOR, J.: Primary intracerebral haemorrhage. A controlled trial of surgical and conservative treatment in 180 unselected cases. Lancet 2, 221-226 (1961).

18. NORLÉN, G.: Die chirurgische Behandlung intracranieller Gefäßmißbildungen. A. Angiome. Handbuch der Neurochirurgie. Hrsg. H. Olivecrona und W. Tönnis, Bd. 4/II, S. 147-206. Berlin-Heidelberg-New York: Springer 1966.

19. OLIVECRONA, H., LADENHEIM, J.: Congenital arteriovenous aneurysms of the carotid and vertebral arterial systems. Berlin: Springer 1957.

20. PATERSON, J. H., MCKISSOCK, W.: A clinical survey of intracranial angiomas with special reference to their mode of progression and surgical treatment: A report of 110 cases. Brain 79, 233-236 (1956).

21. PERRET, G., NISHIOKA, H.: Arteriovenous malformations. An analysis of 545 cases of cranio-cerebral arteriovenous malformations and fistulae reported to the cooperative study. J. Neurosurg. 25, 467-490 (1966).

22. PIA, H. W.: Diagnose und Therapie der Hirnblutungen im Kindesalter. In Leistungen und Ergebnisse der neuzeitlichen Chirurgie, 128-136. Stuttgart: Thieme 1958.

23. PIA, H. W.: Diagnose und Behandlung der spontanen intracerebralen Massenblutungen. Acta Neurochir. 7, 425-439 (1959).

24. PIA, H. W.: The Diagnosis and Treatment of Intraventricular Haemorrhages. Progr. in Brain Research 30, 463-470 (1968).

25. PIA, H. W.: The Operative Treatment of Intracerebral and Intraventricular Hematomas. Acta Neurochir. 27, 149-164 (1972).

26. PIA, H. W.: The Surgical Treatment of Intracerebral Hematomas. In Present Limits of Neurosurgery, Avicenum, 323-328. Prague: Czechoslov. Med. Press 1972.

27. RUSSELL, D. S.: Spontaneous intracranial haemorrhage. Proc. roy. Soc. Med. 47, 689-693 (1954).

28. SCHIEFER, W.: Klinik der intrazerebralen Massenblutungen und spontanen Haematome. In H. Gänshirt: Der Hirnkreislauf, S. 680-714. Stuttgart: Thieme 1972.

29. TÖNNIS, W.: Symptomatologie und Klinik der supratentoriellen arteriovenösen Angiome. 1. Congr. Int de Neurochirurgie, 205-215. Les Editions Acta Med. Belgica 1957.

30. TÖNNIS, W., SCHIEFER, W., WALTER, W.: Signs and symptoms of supratentorial arteriovenous aneurysms. J. Neurosurg. 15, 471-480 (1958).

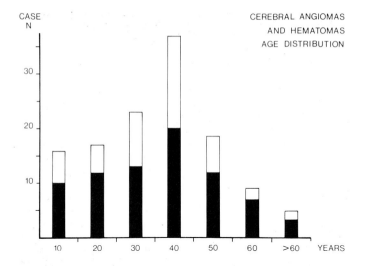

Fig. 1. Age distribution

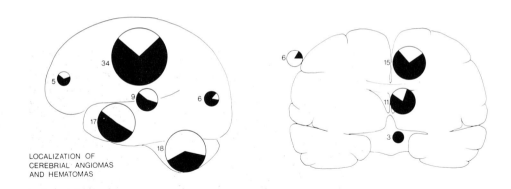

LOCALIZATION OF
CEREBRIAL ANGIOMAS
AND HEMATOMAS

Fig. 2. Localization

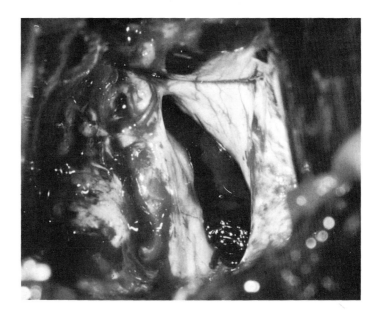

Fig. 3. Intraventricular hematoma (partial ventricular tamponade)

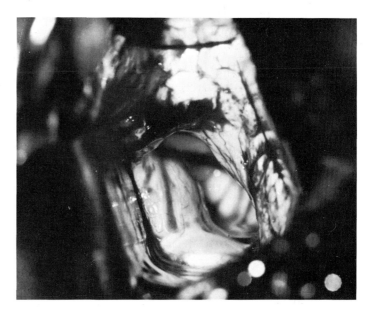

Fig. 4. After washing-out

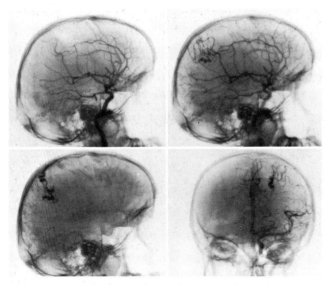

Fig. 5. Angiogram of a right parietal A-V angioma with intracerebral and intraventricular hematomas (Figs. 3, 4)

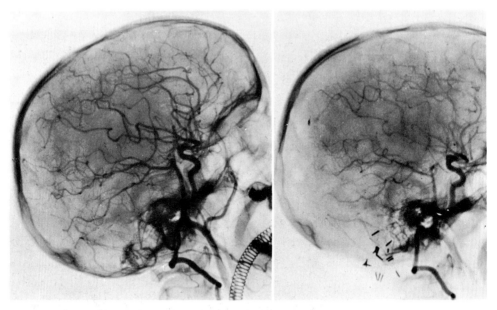

Fig. 6. Angiogram of a cerebellar A-V angioma with an intracerebellar hematoma and a hemorrhage into the ventricle before and after removal and resection

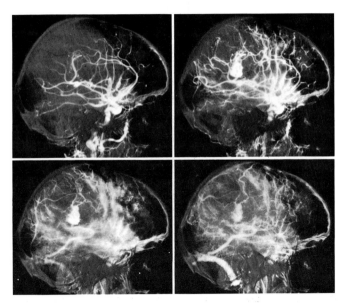

Fig. 7. Angiogram of a deep seated A-V angioma with huge intracerebral hematoma (250 cc)

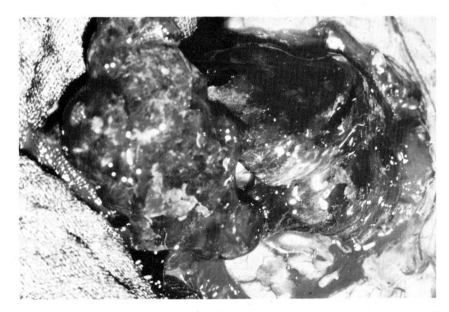

Fig. 8. Same case. After splitting of the cortex

Discussion on Chapter V

PIA: Dr. Kunc has extremely great experience in the ligation of afferent vessels and I regret that he was not able to attend the meeting personally. I think that we all agree that in those angiomas, which are fed by one feeder and which are small, this method is helpful because it brings about total occlusion of the lesion. In other cases, especially in big ones, there is no benefit, and when you see only one or two feeders on total angiography and you have clipped them, control angiography after a short while will new feeding vessels.

BRAUN: I should like to ask some questions related to the following case:

A 24-year-old man had his head pushed while playing soccer. He complained of headache, dizziness and weakness in his left arm and leg. He was brought to a Neurological Clinic, where a lumbar puncture yielded clear spinal fluid. One day later he became drowsy and was transferred to our hospital in a nearly unconscious state with a left hemiplegia. Now the spinal fluid contained blood.

The right carotid arteriogram showed an angioma of the basal ganglia, which was supplied by the anterior choroidal artery and the posterior cerebral artery (Fig. 1). On the vertebral arteriogram the angioma was as large as on the carotid angiogram (Fig. 2). The assumption therefore seemed justified, that the two named arteries were the only blood supply to the angioma. A right temporal craniotomy was performed and the anterior choroidal artery and the posterior cerebral artery were clipped. The patient tolerated the operation well; he was later discharged with a mild residual left hemiparesis and an incomplete leftsided hemianopia.

Control angiography revealed no angioma in the early arterial phases (Fig. 3), but a partial filling in the late arterial phase, apparently brought about by small branches of the middle cerebral artery (Fig.4).

The question must be raised whether this incomplete elimination of the angioma is of any value to the patient at all. It seems to me that so far in this workshop, "partial clipping" has been recommended without due scepticism. Where are the statistics to prove that the occurrence of rebleeding is reduced by this method? In the case Prof. Schürmann described, rebleeding occurred in spite of extensive clipping of feeding vessels.

To avoid craniotomies which are probably rather useless, all the feeding arteries of an angioma must be recognized. Is there any other method such as superselective angiography of the intracerebral branches which will give complete information?

WALTER: With regard to Dr. Braun's question I would draw your attention to 16 cases of our own, in which feeding vessels were clipped. 6 of them suffered from recurrent bleeding and 3 cases which were operated on by clipping of the posterior cerebral artery had a very stormy postoperative course.

SCHÜRMANN: We have had three or four of these cases and operated on 2 of them, who bled. After clipping of the posterior cerebral artery extirpation of a small angioma became possible, because the bleeding into the surrounding tissue gave you a fair demarcation.

PIA: Who has had experience of total extirpation or partial procedures on ventricular and paraventricular angiomas?

JOHNSON: I would like to congratulate Dr. Bushe on his results, especially in those little angiomas that he excised through the ventricle with the aid of the microscope. We have had similar experiences and have excised a few, especially those arising or mainly arising from the choroidal plexus.

FEINDEL: I think that despite all the evidence preoperatively one has surely to assess technical skill and operation team and your own set-up in terms of what is handled. I do not think that any of us, while indicating that one should operate on intraventricular angiomas, would mean that everyone should do it, because these are highly selected to begin with. Most of the ones that we have operated on have presented as hemorrhages. It is very easy to justify an operation in those patients. The difficult one is the patient who may have had a small hemorrhage, be quite well clinically, and you discover the angioma. Then you have to decide what to do. These, I think, if they are fed by reasonably approachable arteries, especially the callosal system, one should operate on although to-day we have to decide whether the patient is willing to accept a degree of hemiparesis. I think our criteria for good operations have to be refined. It is no longer enough just to have a patient surviving.

PERRET: I compliment all my colleagues who have spoken up to the present time. When I was young I also operated on quite a number of intraventricular and paraventricular arteriovenous malformations, but was never able to remove them completely. Most of my removals were just partial removals. In the past ten years I left them alone, and the patients are about as well off.

SANO: If these paraventricular angiomas are treated conservatively, in the long-term follow-up about 50% of them die. This is a much higher mortality than the ordinary mortality of arteriovenous malformations. Therefore we decided to remove these paraventricular angiomas as radically as possible, when it was feasible. Of course this needs a microscope and many hours of surgery. It is also necessary to repeat angiography during the operation many times, because sometimes a part of the lesion may remain.

LUESSENHOP: We have operated on four or five cases, and I think satisfactorily. We use the transventricular approach.

GLEAVE: We have operated on only four of these intraventricular angiomas in Cambridge. They were all done without too much difficulty using the microscope and hypotension.

BURNIE: I have done four intraventricular arteriovenous malformations, two have done well and two have died. So I do not know whether I am going to do many more or not. Earlier to-day you asked for indications for or against operations on a-v malformations. Dr. Luessenhop's observations that a patient, with mild symptoms, intelligent, and afraid, has a right to ask if a cure is available in spite of the very real possibility of a neurological deficit or death shows that he is a very thoughtful and feeling neurosurgeon. And I think that the consideration of the patient should always be foremost. A mildly symptomatic or possibly asymptomatic small, easily accessible a-v malformation is excellent operative training for a young neurosurgeon. As most of you are training younger men, then you can hold their hand during this transition as you help them with their surgery. This sometimes may be an indication for operating on them. And try as hard as you may, the ego of the surgeon, or the expectations of his younger men as to his ability sometimes precipitate actions possibly better left undone. If one does not have the capability for doing the excellent angiography that has been demonstrated here to-day, you have only one thing you can do and that is send the patient somewhere else. And again you cannot let pride get in the way for that can cause another unwise decision. I think it is unnecessary to mention this in front of such an august group, but let us keep it in mind.

LAPRAS: We have tried to cure three paraventricular angiomas but we have never been able to excise them completely. We approached the lesion at the junction of the parietal and occipital lobe transcerebrally, we entered the lateral ventricle, and performed partial clipping.

PIA: All who attended the third Microsurgical Congress in Kyoto were fascinated by the paper of Charles Drake. He reported six or seven cases with a-v malformations of small size, up to that of a cherry, situated in the interpeduncular fossa. He was able to operate upon all these cases and carry out a total excision without any deficit, without any death. I hope that all of us would be able to do the same. I personally have never tried to operate on such really medial angiomas in the interpeduncular fossa. Does anybody else have any experience with these cases?

BUSHE: I would like to draw your attention to the opinion of Dr. Drake, that these angiomas are always located in the subarachnoid space and do not penetrate into the cerebral tissue. It is only because of this that they may be operated upon.

PIA: I think you are speaking about a special type, which is situated extracranially in the subarachnoid space, and this is not the type which was demonstrated this morning by Dr. Jellinger. - Now about the posteriorly located angiomas in the region of the great vein of Galen. Shall we be active or aggressive against these lesions following the experience of Dr. Lapras? As far as cerebellar angiomas are concerned, my experience is that the big ones are very dangerous, but the small ones situated in the cerebellar hemisphere present no problems. May I remind you that Olivecrona in his paper mentioned only one case in which he was able to resect the angioma completely. On all the other cases decompression only was carried out. What change has there been in our attitude towards these lesions during the last ten years?

WALTER: Among 18 cases of angiomas of the posterior fossa of our own, 10 were located in the hemispheres of the vermis. They were all extirpated with good results. But the others, affecting the cord and pons rarely bleed, and produce the symptoms of space-occupying lesions. In these cases a ventriculo-atrial shunt is the method of choice, we have quite a few patients doing fairly well with this treatment.

FEINDEL: I just want to make one point that in some of the vermian angiomas such as I think were described by Dr. Lapras, we have found that there are contributions from the meningeal vessels of the posterior fossa, which go to the torcular and also contribute to the shunt. I think it is important to interrupt these.

PERRET: We have had considerable experience in extirpating angiomas that were easily accessible, that is on the posterior cerebellar surface or on the vermis. But we have not been able to remove completely those on the superior anterior surface of the cerebellum. Now, do you include in this group the arteriovenous malformations that lie on the medulla below the cerebellar tonsils? Do not touch those if they arise from both vertebral arteries. However, recently we had one case of a large arteriovenous malformation overlying the medulla oblongata, the upper cervical cord, and penetrating into the fourth ventricle, which was entirely fed by a branch of the external carotid artery. Once the branch was clipped, we could nearly lift out the arteriovenous malformation.

WALTER: I want to stress the very great value of intraoperative angiography to secure total removal of the malformation.

JOHNSON: We have managed to excise some of the anterior superior angiomas in the cerebellum, and these are the ones that particularly cause trigeminal neuralgia, especially in women during the menstrual period. We operate on them by turning a flap above the sinus and dividing the tentorium so that you can really approach the lesion from the front as well as behind.

LOEW: We had three angiomas located in the cerebellar hemisphere or in the vermis. In one of the cases the malformation extended into the pons. It had bled and had led to a facial paralysis, caused by a vessel loop. I was able to remove the angioma, but I had to leave the intrapontine part with a very small draining vein. The patient is doing well.

LUESSENHOP: It seems that the principal difficulties with the angiomas of the cerebellar hemisphere is that we encounter the venous side before we get to the arterial side. As Mr. Johnson mentioned, this can be helped by going through the tentorium exposing the lesion both below and above the tentorium. I would like to comment on the great vein of Galen malformations. Everyone uses this term because it is an arteriovenous malformation which lies near that area and with good venous drainage it enlarges that vein. There are two types, the first one is an arteriovenous malformation in the brain substance which drains to this vein and dilates it. This should not be called a great vein of Galen malformation. In most instances it is probably not operable. The second type is that in which cerebral arteries do directly communicate with the great vein of Galen and are not within the substance of the brain. This variety is just a fistula external to the brain stem. If it can be proven angiographically, this type should be easily operable.

PENZHOLZ: I think one should only attempt to extirpate totally angiomas in the inferior vermis. I once tried to extirpate totally a malformation located in the superior vermis, and this patient became very handicapped.

PIA: The Giessen team would like to have your opinion about our huge angioma case in which we were encouraged to do hemispherectomy. What experience is there of total extirpation of such malformations? All the arguments in favour of hemispherectomy given by our colleagues pointed to the fact that this patient had an infantile hemiplegia since his fourth or fifth year, and that most probably his speech would not be markedly impaired after the operation.

KOHLMEYER: What were the results of your Amytal-tests?

PIA: We did it bilaterally many times, but because of the enormous shunt and washing out of the Amytal, a valid assessment was impossible.

FEINDEL: We have had the same experience in assessing speech localization in the presence of arteriovenous malformations. Sometimes with small malformations, if you use about double the dose of Amytal you can identify the side of the speech. It would be very difficult to get anything to enter the normal side in such a huge angioma because, as you suggested, it is simply shunted. Even if you inject the right carotid, it would shunt over to the left carotid and the drug does not get into the brain. That is the second reason why you did not really find it useful . If we had to do that case I think we would have approached it in a somewhat similar fashion to the way I showed for the one which was much more favourable, superiorly and anteriorly. We picked off the feeding arteries, distal to the speech area. This would give you only a partial cure, but it could be done without impairing speech. We would have done it under local anaesthesia in order to define the speech area by stimulation.

DJINDJIAN: (commenting on the case of Dr. Zierski) In our experience we have never seen spinal cord angiomas associated with occipital artery feeding vessels. We have found this only in hemangioblastic tumors. In our 107 cases of spinal cord angiomas we have never seen feeding vessels from the occipital artery. In one case we were able to embolize partially an asymptomatic cervical angioma, fed by the occipital artery, but in that case there were no neurological signs, and your case is very exceptional.

BUSHE (to RIECHERT): I congratulate you on your success. I confirm your results from our own cases, that a small exposure tends to produce little neurological deficit, and the use of the operating microscope is of essential importance for otherwise we cannot visualize structures in the depths.

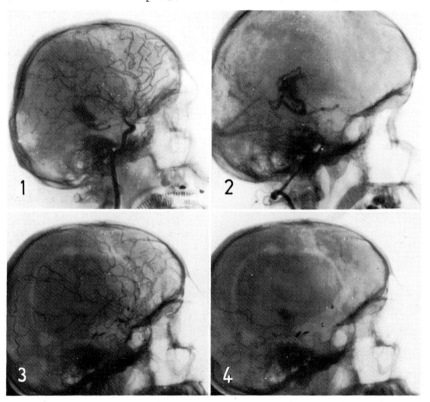

Figs. 1-4. Legends see discussion

Chapter VI

Cryosurgical Treatment

Freezing Arteriovenous Anomalies in the Brain

H. A. D. WALDER

Introduction

The present paper will be concerned with the clinical use of low tem-
peratures in arteriovenous lesions in the brain. The experimental stage
included freezing, not only of normal vessels but also of vascular lesions, i.e. fusiform and saccular aneurysms of the carotid artery and
shunts between the carotid artery and jugular vein in dogs.

To recapitulate briefly: the most important finding was that hemorrhage
will not occur during freezing so long as the following precautions are
adopted:

a) the cryoprobe is held immobile during freezing;
b) the temperature of the cryoprobe must be above freezing point when
   it is withdrawn in order to avoid rupture of the vessel walls.

When these precautions are adopted, no macroscopic injury to the vascular wall has been observed. Microscopy, however, reveals marked
changes: rarefaction of the endothelium in the initial stage, and proliferation of the tunica intima and thrombosis at a subsequent stage.
These two findings provided a rationale for its possible clinical use.

As stated above, an experimental study was done on saccular aneurysms
artificially produced in dogs by implanting a segment of the jugular
vein into the carotid artery. In a large number of these cases thrombosis of the aneurysm was observed, a finding verified by arteriography and microscopy.

The author does not have any clinical experience with saccular aneurysms but he has used the procedure in the treatment of patients with
an arteriovenous aneurysm.

The results of treatment obtained by this method will be discussed in
the light of arteriographic follow-up studies.

Material and Methods

Since 1967, an operation using cryocoagulation has been performed thir-
ty-five times in twenty-seven patients with arteriovenous lesions in
the brain.

As was previously reported by PEETERS (1), intraoperative arteriography was carried out in thirteen cases. This was done in those patients in whom the lesions were located in the deep structures of the brain or in whom the lesions involved the deep structures.

According to the size of the arteriovenous malformation, the cryoprobe was inserted up to a maximum of twenty-five times during a single session.

The temperature was taken down to -100° C for five minutes. On warming, the cryoprobe was altered in position or removed thirty seconds after a temperature of 0° C had been reached. (The radius of the probe was 2.6 mm.).

The results of treatment were evaluated by postoperative arteriography and, in one case, at autopsy (within three weeks of the operation).

Arteriography was not carried out until at least three weeks had elapsed since the operation as experimental studies had shown that thrombosis does not occur until a few weeks later (WALDER 2).

Because of the extent of the lesion, clipping was done in addition to cryocoagulation in five cases.

In twenty-four cases, the indication for surgical treatment was one or more subarachnoid hemorrhages, an intracerebral hematoma being present in four cases.

In three cases, the operation was performed because of epilepsy and progressive deterioration.

In one case, the operation was performed with the patient still in coma as the result of subarachnoid hemorrhage.

The other patients were mentally normal before operation, though nine showed marked symptoms of neurological dysfunction.

The indication for cryocoagulation instead of orthodox surgical treatment was based on the extremely large size of the lesion and/or its location in an area of functional importance in five cases (Table 1, cases 3 and 7; Table 2, cases 5, 9 and 12).

In twelve cases, the indication was the deep-seated location of the lesion (Table 1, cases 10, 11, 13 and 14; Table 2, cases 3, 4, 6, 7, 8, 10, 11 and 13).

On these grounds, sixteen patients from elsewhere were referred to the present author because of alleged inoperability by orthodox surgical procedures.

On account of the simplicity of the technique, cryocoagulation was carried out in the other ten cases, although these patients could probably have been satisfactorily treated by the so-called orthodox procedures.

The age of the patients varied from 12-73 years and included twelve women and fifteen men.

Table 1. Thrombosed cases

Sex	Age	History	Preop.State	Localization	Operation	Postop.State	Postop.Course
1 ♀	49	hemorrhage + coma	coma	a.cer.med.sin	23-3'67 freezing à vue	unchanged coma	died 3 weeks after oper. (embolism)
2 ♀	27	hemorrhage + coma	conscious	a.cer.post.sin	19-9-'67 freezing à vue + extirp.	conscious	uneventful
3 ♀	73	hemorrhage + coma	conscious	a.cer.ant.sin	1-11'68 freezing à vue	conscious	uneventful
4 ♂	9	hemorrhage + coma	conscious	a.calloso marg. dextra	22-8'69 freezing à vue	conscious	uneventful
5 ♀	42	hemorrhage 2 x + coma	conscious	a.cer.med.ant. dextra haematoma	2-11'69 freezing à vue	conscious	uneventful
6 ♂	41	hemorrhage 2 x + subcoma	conscious hemiparesis	a.cer.med. + post.dextra haematoma	4-12'69 freezing à vue	conscious hemiparesis	uneventful hemiparesis
7 ♀	43	hemorrhage 2 x + coma + epilepsy	conscious hemiparesis	a.cer.ant. dextra	7-8'70 16-9'67 freezing + clipping	conscious	unchanged uneventful hemiparesis
8 ♂	46	hemorrhage + coma	conscious hemiparesis	a.cer.med.sin. haematoma	3-12'70 freezing à vue	conscious	uneventful hemiparesis
9 ♂	39	hemorrhage + coma	conscious	a.cer.med.sin. + haematoma	4-2-'71 freezing à vue	conscious	uneventful
10 ♂	36	hemorrhage 2 x	conscious	a.cer.post.sin.	29-3'71 freezing + perop.art. contr. (a.verte-bralis)	conscious no neurol. sympt.	uneventful

Table 1 (continued)

Sex	Age	History	Preop.State	Localization	Operation	Postop.State	Postop.Course
11 ♂	39	hemorrhage	conscious	a.cer.med.	2-4-'71 26-4-'71 freezing + perop.art. control.	conscious no neurol. sympt.	uneventful
12 ♀	39	epileptic seizures	conscious	a.cer.med.dextra	18-1'72 freezing + clipping	conscious no neurol. sympt.	uneventful
13 ♀	20	hemorrhage	conscious	a.cer.ant.sin.	10-8-'72 freezing à vue	conscious	uneventful
14 ♂	31	hemorrhage	conscious hemianops	a.cer.post. dextra	11-1'73 freezing à vue	conscious neurol.state unchanged.	uneventful

Table 2. Cases with remnants

Sex	Age	History	Preop.State	Localization	Operation	Postop.State	Postop.Course	Remnants
1 ♀	15	hemorrhage + coma	conscious	a.cer.ant. dextra	24-5'68 freezing à vue	conscious	uneventful	50 %
2 ♂	37	hemorrhage + coma	conscious	a.lenticulo str.dextra	14-10'68 freezing à vue	conscious	uneventful	60 %
3 ♀	41	hemorrhage 2 x + sub- coma	conscious + hemiparesis dextra	a.cer.med. + post.sin.	3-10'69 freezing + perop.contr.	conscious + hemiparesis	uneventful hemiparesis improved	10 %
4 ♂	39	hemorrhage 4 x + coma	conscious	a.cer.peri- callosa sin.	21-1'70 stereotact	conscious no neurol.	recurrence of hemorrhage 13-5'71	40 %

No.	Sex	Age	Presentation	Neurological status	Localization	Date / procedure	Post-op status	Course	%
5	♂	29	hemorrhage 2 x + coma	conscious hemianopt.	a.cer.ant. + med.sin.	13-1-'70 clipping + freezing	conscious hemianopt.	uneventful	50 %
6	♂	15	hemorrhage	conscious	a.cer.pericall. sin.	17-2-'71 27-3-'71 freezing + perop.contr.	conscious no neurol. sympt.	recurrence of hemorrhage	60 %
7	♀	24	hemorrhage 3 x + coma	hemiparesis hemihypaes-thesia hemianopt.	a.lent.str. dextra bas.gangl.	1-3-'72 freezing + perop. contr.	conscious neurol.un-changed	uneventful	10 %
8	♀	25	hemorrhage 1 x + coma	hemiparesis	a.cer.med. a.cer.ant. thalamus	freezing + perop.contr. 13-3-'72	conscious hemiparesis	uneventful	50 %
9	♀	21	hemorrhage 2 x	conscious	a.cer.media d. a.cer.pericall. d. a.cer.post.d.	16-12-'71 16-3-'72 freezing + clipping perop.contr.	conscious	uneventful	10 %
10	♂	42	hemorrhage 5 x	conscious	a.chor.ant.sin.	10-7-1972 freezing + perop.contr.	conscious	uneventful	40 %
11	♂	36	hemorrhage 2 x	conscious hemiparesis hemianaes-thesia	a.chor.ant.d. a.cer.port.d.	6-12-1972 29-1-1973 freezing + perop.contr.	conscious	uneventful	30 %
12	♂	48	epileptic seizures	conscious	a.cer.med. et post.sin.	18-1-1973 freezing + clipping	conscious	recurrence 5-10-1973+	
13	♂	12	hemorrhage + coma	conscious	A.thal.striat. dextra	12-1-'73 stereotactic + perop.contr.	conscious conscious	uneventful uneventful	10 % 30 %

Results

The arteriovenous lesion was totally eliminated (Figs.1, 2) in fourteen of twenty-seven cases treated surgically (Table 1).

The thirteen cases in which complete thrombosis did not occur, showed that between 10 to 60 percent of the total preoperative extent of the arteriovenous malformation was left (Table 2).

Twenty-six patients had an uneventful postoperative course, and one woman died from a pulmonary embolism originating from thrombosis in the right leg within three weeks of the operation.

Nine patients showed symptoms of neurological dysfunction before operation. There was a marked improvement in the neurological status during the postoperative period in three cases, the status quo ante being observed in five cases, and a slight worsening being present in one case.

Recurrent hemorrhage was seen in three of the cases in whom total thrombosis had not occurred, the hemorrhage terminating in death in one case.

The other two patients were admitted to other hospitals and surgical treatment was successful in them. It should be pointed out that these two patients as well as the third patient (a child) had been initially referred to the hospital of the author because the arteriovenous lesion was believed to be inoperable.

It should be stressed that, in the five patients considered to be inoperable because of the location and extent of the lesion, the malformation was totally eliminated in two and partially in three cases.

In those patients in whom the lesion was regarded as inoperable because of its deep-seated location, it was totally eliminated in four and partially in eight cases.

In the other ten patients, the malformation was totally eliminated in eight and partially in two cases.

Comment

Closer examination of these results suggests that the number of failures in the sense of partial elimination in thirteen out of twenty-seven cases should be considered unduly large.

This treatment therefore was successful in six cases, and partial success was obtained in eleven out of seventeen cases whose condition apparently was not amenable to orthodox surgical treatment.

It should be pointed out that, whereas the proliferation of the endothelial tissue observed in the experimental studies will not prevent recurrent hemorrhage (Table 2, cases 4, 6 and 11), partial elimination of the lesion did reduce the so-called steal effect in other cases.

This reduction was revealed clinically as well as by postoperative arteriography (Fig. 3).

Another good point was the fact that the postoperative course was uneventful in twenty-six cases.

This holds good for the general clinical course as well as for the neurological status.

The inadequate number of histological specimens available makes it hard to account for the failures but the present author believes that the causes in those cases in which the lesions were extensive and deep-seated were twofold.

To begin with, a very rapid rate of blood flow is an adverse factor as part of the blood vessel will be inadequately cooled because of the unduly large supply of heat.

In addition, the majority of arteriovenous lesions are slightly encapsulated so that the cryoprobe cannot come into adequate contact with the abnormal vessels as the congerie, in a manner of speaking, thrust ahead of the cryoprobe which thus does not come to be situated in the midst of the abnormal vessels. This was occasionally observed in superficial arteriovenous lesions in which, however, this drawback can readily be overcome.

It is much more difficult, however, to determine whether this is so in deep-seated lesions as the only method of observation available in these cases is intraoperative arteriography.

This view is supported by the satisfactory results (total elimination in eight out of ten cases) obtained using cryocoagulation in those lesions which, because of their relatively convenient location and limited extent could also have been treated by orthodox surgical procedures.

S u m m a r y

Summarizing, it can be stated that wider experience has shown that cryocoagulation as a method of treatment in patients with arteriovenous lesions does not fully come up to the expectations based on experimental studies.

In particular, the number of failures in so-called inoperable lesions (viz. in eleven out of seventeen cases), was unduly large.

The author therefore believes that this method of treatment has failed to provide a solution to the problem and that the procedure is still subject to considerable limitations.

On the other hand, the method does represent a further advance in the search for a solution to the problem of treatment in these cases.

The hazards involved in this form of treatment are obviously less serious than they are in orthodox surgery.

References

1. PEETERS, F. L. M., WALDER, H. A. D., VROOMEN, J. G. H.: Intraoperative zerebrale Angiographie. Fortschritte auf dem Gebiete der Röntgenstrahlen und der nuklear Medizin. Band 112, Heft 5, 615-621 (1970).

2. WALDER, H. A. D., JASPAR, H. H. J., MEIJER, E.: Application of cryotherapy in cerebro-vascular anomalies (an experimental and clinical study). Psychiatria, Neurologia, Neurochirurgia, 73, 471-480 (1970).

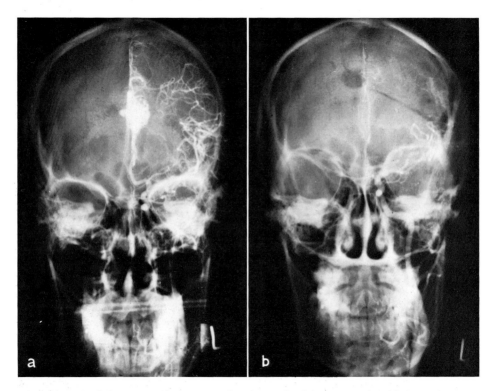

Fig. 1 a and b. Arteriovenous lesion of the a. pericallosa sin., pre- and postoperative

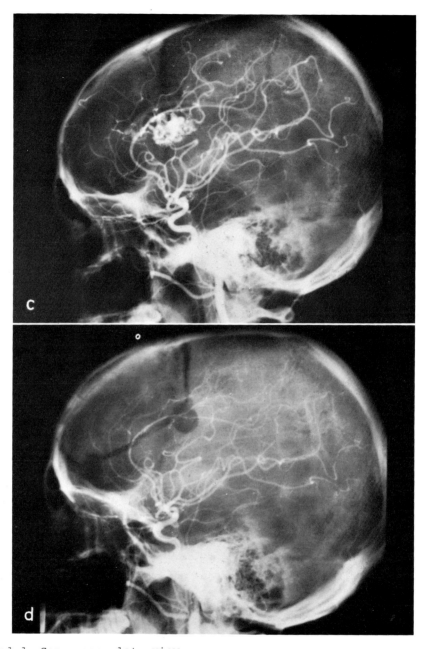

Fig. 1 c and d. Same case, lat. view

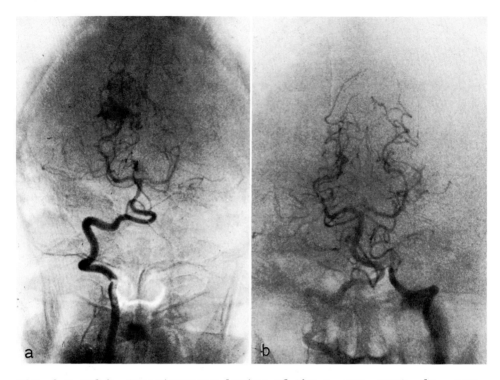

Fig. 2 a and b. Arteriovenous lesion of the a. cer. post. dx., pre-
and postoperative

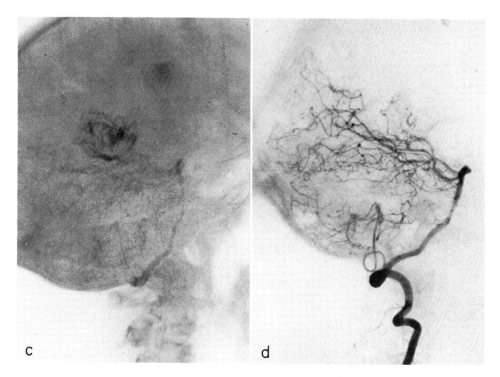

Fig. 2 c and d. Same case before and after cryocoagulation

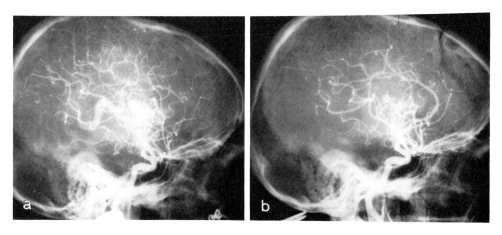

Fig. 3 a. Status before cryosurgery of arteriovenous lesion in the region of the lenticulostriate artery. Stealing has considerably reduced the filling of the anterior cerebral artery

Fig. 3 b. Status after cryosurgery. Partial elimination of the lesion. Stealing no longer occurs; adequate filling of anterior cerebral artery

Discussion on Chapter VI

GLEAVE: I have used cryosurgery in only one case. Most of the technical discussion here has been on the difficulties provided by very large angiomas. I have encountered difficulty in actually finding three small angiomas where there was no clot cavity to guide me to the site. The case I want to demonstrate was a 59-year-old man with a small arteriovenous malformation. This was his second bleed, the first having occurred 2o years ago when he was 39, and he then remained reasonably well with a mild left hemiparesis. No angiogram had been done at the time of the first hemorrhage. I anticipated, looking at the angiograms, that I might very well find difficulty in finding this angioma by orthodox surgery. Inspired by the work of Dr. Walder, I wondered whether it might not be possible to do this stereotactically using the cryoprobe. The temperature was taken down to minus 80 degrees in two positions for three minutes at a time. I was somewhat disappointed 3 months later to see no apparent change in the arteriovenous malformation. On very close inspection possibly a few of the very fine vessels had disappeared but the actual shunt almost looked to be quicker than it had been. A year later, however, with no intervening occurrence to suggest any thrombolic or hemorrhagic episode, the arteriovenous malformation had disappeared. Whether this was due to cryosurgery or whether it was due to natural phenomenon, I do not know for certain, but suspect the former.

WALDER: I am sorry, I do not have such a late control angiogram. Six months after surgery, we have seen that an a-v malformation got smaller, but there has been no total disappearance. I think the whole background of this treatment is that you damage the vessel wall, and this leads to thrombosis.

LOEW: I have had some contact with Dr. Walder's patients. I feel that his conclusions are too negative. He is too critical in emphasizing the negative side of the picture. His treatment had no deleterious effect on his patients; some of them were cured, who in usual terms were regarded as inoperable. I think this method is useful.

JOHNSON: I share Dr. Loew's opinion. An inoperable case which has been cured is a case gained. That sort of case is extremely impressive to the patient, to his relatives, and to the surgeon, but gets lost in the statistics.

PIA: It was my original plan to get Dr. Ambrose to come to us. But we are very happy that Dr. Johnson and Dr. Feindel will speak about their experiences with the EMI scanner in diagnosing a-v malformations.

JOHNSON: With the EMI-scanner sections are taken in that plane in which the old neuropathologists used to cut the brain. I think it is a plane of section that really gives you more information about the brain than the usual sagittal and coronal planes that we are so familiar with. The scan can be repeated at intervals, daily if you like, and you can watch the progress of the lesion.

FEINDEL: I agree with Mr. Johnson that the EMI-scanner brings a remarkable amount of information to the diagnosis of intracerebral hematomas

of all kinds. This example from Dr. Ambrose's series shows the intracerebral clot somewhat deep in the left side but not breaking through
either to the ventricle or to the surface. As Mr. Johnson has shown,
the geography of the hematoma can be seen for the first time so that
if you look at this and the relationship of the hematoma to the brain
structure, you can make a rational decision as to whether operate or
not. You can distinguish the deep capsular hematoma, the small one from
the superficial one, the temporal lobe hematoma (Fig. 1). You can decide to put a burr-hole where the hematoma comes most superficially.
A very remarkable example of Dr. Ambrose's which we were reviewing last
summer was a patient who had a small a-v angioma in the posterior part
of the left temporal horn with an intraventricular hemorrhage, and it
is really thrilling to see the intraventricular hemorrhages. It is like
a concrete cast of the ventricle so that it gives you the position, the
topography, the presence or not of intraventricular hematomas, and
whether there is a ventricular shift all on the same picture. As Mr.
Johnson says, it is the vesalian horizontal section of the brain which
the surgeon finds much more useful than the standard antroposterior or
lateral films of radiology. Those of course, we sometimes forget, produce a foreshortened effect bringing a three dimensional round head
into the flat plane to which we have become accustomed. In this section of the head there is no distortion of the anatomical relation-
ships. Now curiously enough the first patient that we did in Canada
on the EMI-scanner had this a-v malformation. A young teacher who was
watching television suddenly became numb and paralysed down his left
side with very little headache and preservation of consciousness. We
felt that he probably had had a hemorrhage or an infarct. The angiogram (Fig. 2) was done at an outside hospital and then next we did his
EMI-scan (Fig. 3). This shows in the upper right part two features.
One is the slight increase in the density, which we took to be a small
hematoma, and then you see a rather large area of low density which we
have come to recognize as edema. Then you see a little something in
the midline that is probably a bit of a hematoma. Now we elected to
wait on him rather than operate thinking that a good deal of this was
swelling and not very much was hematoma. Because the malformation was
in the leg area we tried to avoid going in acutely. This proved to be
reasonable. A great deal of his hemiplegia recovered over the next few
weeks and we went in and closed off this single feeding artery without
trying to remove the angioma. He showed the striking phenomenon Dr.
Walder mentioned just a few minutes ago, that by reducing the steal
syndrome the weakness of his foot improved within 24 hours, which I
think indicates the mechanism of it. In summary, we have done 300 cases
now with the Montreal scanner. Dr. Ambrose has something over 800 cases.
I think the experience has been that the acute hematoma gives a high
density picture. The reason for this is still not clear. It is probably
either the calcium or the iron which has a high atomic number and comes
out at a high density. Secondly, you get low density edema around a
clot which provides you with some evidence, surgically, as to where to
go. It certainly gives you a great deal of information as to the dis-
position, the size and the surgical location of the hematoma. In the
large angiomas you sometimes see a little irregularity on the scan,
even without hemorrhage, and if you use the Ambrose technique of intravenous injection of contrast medium, you get enhancement of the vessels so that you do see some of the shadows of the vessels standing
out to give you the outline of the angioma. Of course, this is nothing
compared with the radiological picture, but it is useful. The other
point is that it is quite easy to identify an infarct from a hematoma,
and this is of great importance. So combining the EMI-scanner with angiography for the acute cases should give us all a very much better
rationale for approaching acute hematomas both in hypertensive cases,
aneurysms, and in a-v malformations.

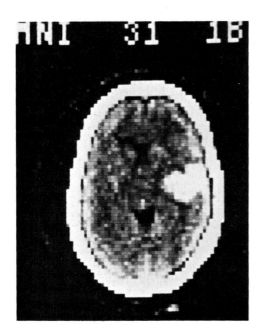

Fig. 1. EMI scan of the Montreal Neurological Institute series showing spontaneous intracerebral hematoma in the right temporal region. Note the well-defined outline of the hemorrhage and its extension to the surface of the grey matter, at which point it was readily evacuated during operation. The patient's left hemiparesis began to improve on the day after operation

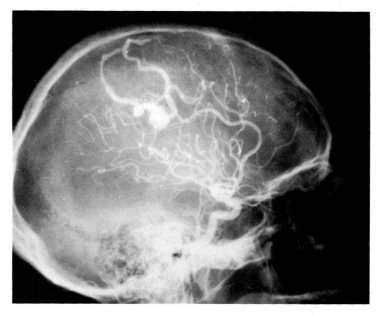

Fig. 2. A small angioma situated deeply in the mesial fronto-parietal cortex of the motor region and fed by a large branch of the anterior cerebral artery. The patient had a sudden onset of left-sided sensory and motor paralysis

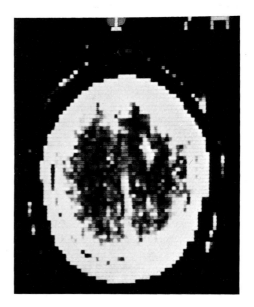

Fig. 3. EMI scan on the same patient. The bright area in the anterior part of the right hemisphere, just to the right of the midline indicates a small hematoma and around this there is a darker area indicating edema. This was the first patient in the Montreal Neurological Institute EMI scan series

Chapter VII
Artificial Embolization

Artificial Embolization of Inoperable Arteriovenous Malformations

A. J. LUESSENHOP

I n t r o d u c t i o n

During the past fourteen years we have been treating certain inoperable cerebral arteriovenous malformations by embolization. Most of
these patients required several procedures via both the carotid and
vertebral circulations. In some the procedures were staged for the same
artery over intervals of a few weeks to one year. In total, we have
performed 94 procedures on 55 patients utilizing over 3,000 emboli.
During this period approximately 250 cases have been seen by our service. A greater number were treated by direct surgical excision and a
few were considered untreatable by any method we know today.

The anatomical and physiological bases for artificial embolization have
been described in previous publications (LUESSENHOP, 1, 2) and are now
well known. Therefore, this will not be discussed here. Our indications
for artificial embolization are now quite rigid. We select only those
patients with enlarged arterial channels leading directly to the lesion
from the cervical arteries. The lesions must be inoperable because of
size or location in a critical area. The patients must be symptomatic
with a history of a single or repeated bleeding, intractable head pain,
or a neurological deficit with or without associated hydrocephalus.
Seizures as a sole manifestation of smaller lesions is not an indication of embolization by our present criteria. Embolization preliminary
to surgical excision has been utilized in seven patients. This is most
useful when enlarged draining veins obscure the deeper feeding arteries,
as in the Sylvian fissure or the posterior portions of the cerebellar
hemispheres (Figs. 1, 2, 3, 4).

Because of multiple collateral channels leading to the lesion it is not
anticipated that embolization will totally eliminate all sites of artery to vein communication. We have achieved total elimination of a
lesion, proven by angiography one year post embolization, in only one
case. The objectives of the procedure are to reduce the flow through
the fistulas, thereby increasing the flow to the surrounding brain,
and reduce the size of the draining veins which compress the brain or
cause hydrocephalus by obstruction within the ventricular system. Also,
by reducing the sizes of the feeding arteries, headache may be relieved
particularly in the posterior cerebral artery territories. As long as
some portion of the lesion persists, the potential for bleeding remains.

Technique

The surgical technique utilizing large catheters introduced directly
into the common carotid artery for embolization of the internal and
external carotid systems and into the subclavian artery for embolization via the vertebrobasilar system has been described in previous
publications (1, 2). We have continued to use silastic spheres contain-
ing metallic markers. The technique has been modified using transcuta-
neous catheters and other forms of material for the emboli, particularly for vascular lesions in the external carotid territory and spinal
cord arteriovenous malformations (3, 4). These catheters techniques
preclude the use of very large emboli usually necessary for cerebral
lesions, therefore, we have used these only for spinal cord arteriovenous malformations. It is now possible to monitor the procedure in the
operating room utilizing fluoroscopic imaging and fewer polaroid films
are necessary. The procedure in a typical case is shown in Figs. 5, 6,
7 and 8.

Results

The followup for our cases ranges from 2 months to 14 years averaging
4.5 years. The immediate angiographic effectiveness of embolization
varied from case to case but in all cases it was carried to the maximum
safe limits of the procedure. For purposes of followup evaluation, we
excluded two patients in whom the embolization was not completed for
technical reasons, a patient in whom the lesion was totally obliterated, 8 patients who later underwent surgical excision, and 7 patients
who at the time of embolization were markedly deteriorated with severe
neurological deficits from previous hemorrhages and hydrocephalus. In
the latter group we were able to reverse the deficit and restore the
patient to an active life on one occasion only.

In our experience the major clinical manifestations including headaches,
seizures, neurological deficit and bleeding are independent. Therefore,
we have evaluated the results according to each of these symptoms.

Headache

Fifteen patients in whom intractable headache was a major symptom have
been followed for 4 months to 7.5 years averaging 4 years. Significant
and persisting relief of this symptom was achieved in 12 of the 15.
In the 3 failures there were major functional components. Two were
chronically depressed and the third had severe hysterical manifestations. In most the lesions were in the posterior cerebral artery territory producing a migranoid syndrome and in others there were major
contributions from dural and scalp arteries.

Neurological Deficit

Twelve patients, who during months or years prior to embolization had
focal neurological deficits, have been followed from one to 7.5 years
averaging 3.5 years. Two had obstructive hydrocephalus requiring ven-
triculoatrial shunts and the relative contribution of this to their
symptomotology was difficult to access. In 8 of the 12 the progression
of the deficit arrested and their neurological status remained stable

for the duration of followup ranging from 1 to 4.5 years averaging 3
years. In 3 patients the neurological deficit improved substantially
for 3 years in two and 7 years in one. This latter patient, with a
large parietal lobe lesion, deteriorated again after 7 years, but improved with repeat embolization to eliminate collateral contribution
from the posterior cerebral artery. Only in one patient was embolization ineffective. This patient died elsewhere from unrelated causes 3
and a half years later. Whether or not she developed hydrocephalus is
not known.

Seizures

Nineteen patients who had seizures have been followed for 6 months to
10 years averaging 4 years. In 8 of these the number of seizures was
greatly reduced and in 3 there have been no recurrent seizures. However, in the remaining 11 there was no obvious effect from the embolization and one patient had her first seizure following the embolization. Improved anticonvulsant medication could account for the improvement seen in 8 of the 19 patients.

Subarachnoid or Intracerebral Hemorrhage

There were 21 patients who had one or more hemorrhage prior to embolization. Followup in these patients ranged from 2 months to 14 years
averaging 5 years. In 11 of the 21 there were documented recurrent hemorrhages following embolization. In 5 of these the hemorrhage was fatal
but autopsies in 2 showed that the source of the hemorrhage was an associated saccular aneurysm. Four patients, who had never had a hemorrhage prior to embolization, had one following the procedure. In 3 this
occurred within a few days after embolization.

Discussion and Comments

From our experience with artificial embolization covering fourteen
years it is evident that the procedure is safe in selected patients
with inoperable lesions. When performed to the maximum capability of
the procedure, effective relief of associated headache can be achieved
and a progressive neurological deficit can be stabilized and frequently reversed. Occasionally, it may be possible to reverse a profound
neurological damage. Hydrocephalus frequently occurs with the very large
lesions and should be treated simultaneously by a shunting procedure.
It is unlikely that artificial embolization reduces the seizure potential or the likelihood of recurrent hemorrhage.

Summary

Fifty-five patients with large inoperable cerebral arteriovenous malformations have undergone 94 separate embolization procedures and followed from 2 months to 14 years averaging 4.5 years. It was possible
to stabilize and reverse focal or neurological deficits in most of the
patients and eliminate associated headache. However, there was no prov-
en effect on the potential for recurrent seizures and recurrent spontaneous bleeding. Only rarely is it possible to totally eliminate a
a lesion by artificial embolization.

References

1. LUESSENHOP, A. J.: Artificial embolization for cerebral arteriovenous malformations. In: Krayenbühl, H., Maspes, P. E., Sweet, W.H.
   (eds.): Progr. neurol. Surg. Vol. 3, pp. 320-362. Basel: Karger and
   Chicago: Year Book 1969.

2. LUESSENHOP, A. J., KACHMANN, R., SHEVLIN, W., FERRO, A. A.: Clinical
   evaluation of embolization in the management of large cerebral arteriovenous malformations. J. Neurosurg. $\underline{23}$, 400-417 (1965).

3. DOPPMAN, J. L., DICHIRO, G., OMMAYA, A. K.: Percutaneous embolization of spinal cord arteriovenous malformations. J. Neurosurg. $\underline{34}$,
   48-55 (1971).

4. DJINDJIAN, R., COPHIGNON, J., THÉRON, J., MERLAND, J. J., HOUDART,
   R.: Embolization by superselective arteriography from the femoral
   route in neuroradiology. Review of 60 cases. 1. Technique, indications, complications. Neurorad. $\underline{6}$, 20-26 (1973).

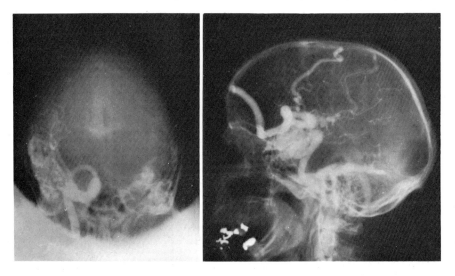

Fig. 1. A large lesion of the temporal lobe and Sylvian fissure difficult for surgical excision

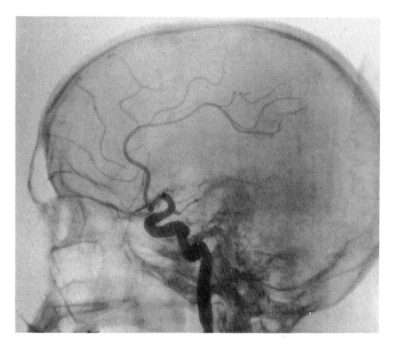

Fig. 2. Same case as Fig. 1 after one 3.5 mm embolus blocks the terminal middle cerebral artery

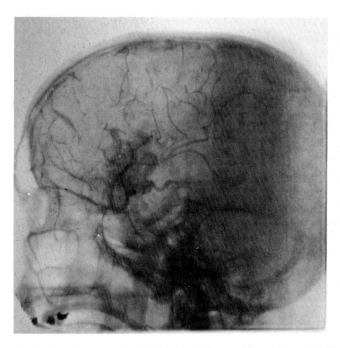

Fig. 3. Same case as Fig. 1 showing collateral circulation to the Sylvian territory via the anterior cerebral artery

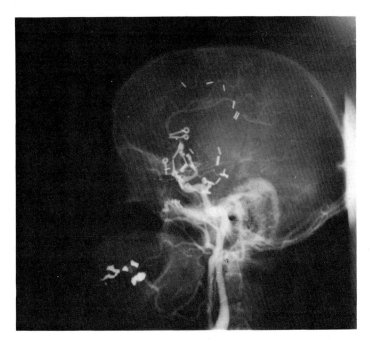

Fig. 4. Same case as Fig. 1 after complete excision of the lesion without neurological deficit

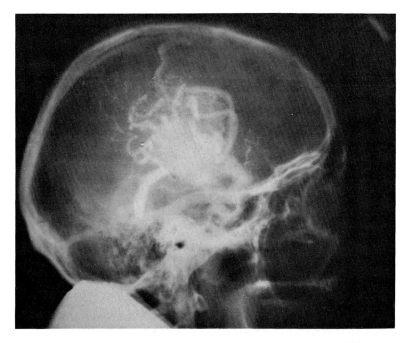

Fig. 5. A large inoperable arteriovenous malformation in the middle
cerebral artery territory of the dominant hemispheres suitable for
embolization

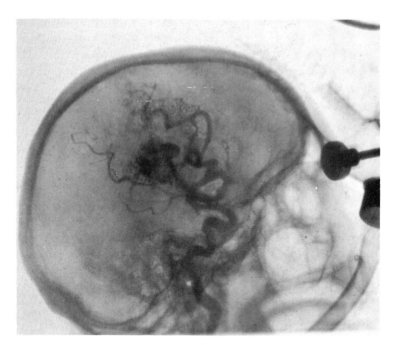

Fig. 6. Same case as Fig. 5 showing reduction of the lesion after 15
2.5 and 3.0 mm silastic emboli

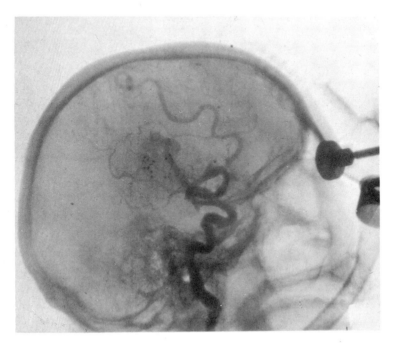

Fig. 7. Same case as Fig. 5 after 22 emboli

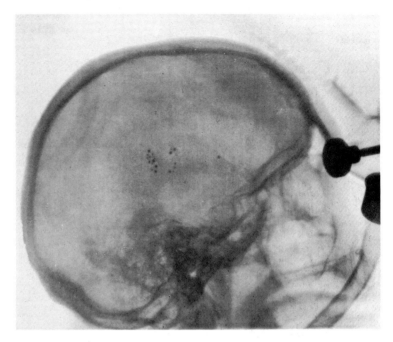

Fig. 8. Same case as Fig. 5 showing final position of emboli

Experiences in the Use of Artificial Embolization as a Method of Treating Cerebral Angiomas

T. Tzonos, R. Bergleiter and F. Pampus

In 1960, LUESSENHOP and SPENCE (7) described a method of artificial embolization of inoperable cerebral angiomas. In 1965, LUESSENHOP et al. (9) published the results of treatment of fifteen such cases. They used steel spheres covered with silastic and having a diameter of one to six mm, as emboli. These spheres were introduced retrogradely via the external carotid artery into the internal carotid artery or directly into the vertebral artery. Since then, more literature has been published on the subject. ROBLES and CARRASCO-ZANINI successfully treated four patients with cerebral and spinal angiomas using muscle emboli. DOPPMAN et al. have attempted the procedure on five patients using steel sheres, pieces of muscle and Gelfoam. This method has also been used in the treatment of haemangiomas of the face (6). DJINDJIAN et al. have been very active in this field and in 1972 reported having done over thirty percutaneous embolizations, using different materials.

Their cases included cerebral, dura and spinal cord angiomas as well as tumors having a rich vascular supply. In an earlier paper, we discussed three cases and presented our initial findings on the treatment of patients with cerebral angiomas (10).

We have performed artificial embolization on ten patients having intracerebral arteriovenous malformations and on four patients with angiomas of the dura. There have been no deaths. Two patients showed marked neulological deficit. The result in all other patients varied from very good to good.

A typical example is given below: Since the age of 16 a 42-year-old woman had had attacks of leftsided headache and loss of orientation, though there were no abnormal neurological findings. Arteriograms showed a very large arteriovenous malformation of the left hemisphere extending up to the midline (Figs. 1 - 3). Figs. 4 - 6 show the state following after embolization. One year later the patient felt well, and there were no abnormal clinical findings.

As the result of these personal experiences, we have found the following method to be the best.

Embolization should begin with the percutaneous selective catheterization as high as possible of the main vessel supplying the angioma (the internal carotid, the external carotid, the occipital or the vertebral artery). The advantage of this procedure is that it can be repeated and that most patients tolerate it well. The disadvantage, on the other hand, is that one can only pass a relatively narrow-bore catheter percutaneously and can therefore introduce only a few emboli by injection as a greater number usually block the catheter lumen. The result is that many injections using large amounts of fluid become necessary. This too, has its limitations. The use of the small 1 mm emboli diminishes the risk incurred when the blood flow is tested. The success of embolization is dependent upon the strength of the flow. This can only be tested during the procedure, as the flow alone is responsible for the carriage of emboli to the angioma. We have found that it is better to use small emboli so that the whole angioma can be filled. The embolization of a major vessel leading to an angioma entails the risk that a collateral blood supply will immediately be formed from other vessels which had not previously been affected.

If, after repeated cerebral embolization, the blood flow proves to be sufficient, then the external carotid or vertebralis artery can be exposed at a later procedure allowing larger emboli to be introduced directly through a wider catheter. This necessitates the ligation of the vessel which precludes further embolization.

The total obliteration of an angioma by this method is, in practice, not possible. However, extensive embolization can markedly reduce the shunt, thus increasing the blood supply to the brain as well as decreasing the danger of rupture and the strain on the heart.

The success of embolization can be assessed through repeated angiograms. Here too, however, there are limits to the amount of dye which can be used and on how well patients tolerate this procedure.

We have often found that the spheres go astray en route to the angioma, landing in other areas, in homolateral or contralateral vessels. (See also LUESSENHOP et al., ROSENBLUTH et al.) There seems to be no relationship between the size of the spheres or their covering (i.e. with or without silastic) and their tendency to wander.

Aside from the blood flow through the angioma, another factor which determines the path of the emboli is the state of the overall circulation at the moment of the injection. This can mean, for example, that after injection into the internal carotid artery, emboli may be carried towards the heart. In some cases it was possible to mobilize such emboli through suction or repositioning of the patient's head. We have also observed that some emboli changed their position after days or weeks and moved towards the angioma, but that other balls in the healthy hemisphere had been carried towards the periphery of the middle cerebral territory.

The effect of embolization is almost entirely a mechanical one. Secondary thrombosis plays a subsiduary role. In one of our own cases which we had embolized with 53 one mm spheres 4 weeks before extirpation of the angioma we found in 30 serial sections only 4 small vessels which showed thrombosis.

The extracerebral angiomas have a tendeny to form a collateral circulation most quickly, as they receive their blood supply from many sources. Such angiomas must therefore be embolized more frequently and within a shorter time span. We recommend that embolization begins at the periphery, and works inwards to as close as possible to the main trunk, in order to prevent the formation of a collateral circulation through more distal vessels.

Despite all this, embolization is not enough in every case. Even if the presenting symptoms have improved, sometimes after the lapse of months,

207

complete success is only possible through surgical intervention and the ligation of still patent vessels, for example from the perforating vessels of the occipital bone or the tentorial artery. It may also be possible to increase the blood flow through the angioma by first ligating the easily accessible branches, thereby increasing the chances of embolizing the inaccessible branches.

The risk that emboli will travel into uninvolved and important vessels is impossible to influence or prevent. Nevertheless we have illustrated and discussed these methods which present a feasible way of treating otherwise inoperable cases. Until now, attempts to influence the course of emboli through the use of extracranial magnets have been a failure (YODH et al. (5)).

S u m m a r y

We have performed artificial embolization on 10 patients with intra-cerebral arteriovenous malformations and on 4 patients with angiomata of the dura. 2 patients showed marked neurological deficits. The result in all other patients varied from very good to good.

The embolization should begin using the percutaneous catheter technique. The use of small 1 mm emboli diminishes the risk incurred when the blood flow is assessed. The filling of the angioma with emboli avoids the danger of the development of a later collateral blood supply. The effect of embolization is almost completely a mechanical one. Consequent thrombosis plays a secondary role.

R e f e r e n c e s

1. DJINDJIAN, R., HOUDART, R., COPHIGNON, J., HURTH, M., COMOY, J.: Premiers essais d'embolisation par voie fémorale de fragments de muscle dans un cas d'angiome médullaire et dans un cas d'angiome alimenté par la carotide externe. Rev. Neurolog. (Paris) 120, 119-130 (1971).

2. DJINDJIAN, R., COPHIGNON, J., THÉRON, J., MERLAND, J. J., HOUDART, R.: L'embolisation en neuro-radiologie vasculaire. Nouv. Pres. Med. 33, 2153-2158 (1972).

3. DOPPMAN, J. L., DI CHIRO, G., OMMAYA, A. K.: Obliteration of spinal-cord arteriovenous malformation by percutaneous embolisation. Lancet (1968 I) 477.

4. DOPPMAN, J.L., DI CHIRO, G., OMMAYA, A.K.: Percutaneous embolisation of spinal cord arteriovenous malformations. J. Neurosurg. 34, 48-55 (1971).

5. YODH, S. B., PIERCE, N. T., WEGGEL, R. J., MONTGOMERY, D. B.: A new magnet system for "intravascular navigation". Med. biol. Engng. 6, 143-147 (1968).

6. LONGACRE, J. J., BENTON, C., UNTERTHINER, R. A.: Treatment of facial haemangioma by intravascular embolisation with silicone spheres. Plast. Reconstruct. Surg. 50, 618-621 (1972).

7. LUESSENHOP, A. J., SPENCE, W. T.: Artificial embolisation of cerebral arteries. Report of use in a case of arteriovenous malformation. J. Amer. med. Ass. 172, 1153-1155 (1960).

8. LUESSENHOP, A. J., GIBBS, M., VELASQUEZ, A. C.: Cerebrovascular response to emboli. Observations in patients with arteriovenous malformations. Arch. Neurol. (Chicago) 7, 264-274 (1962).

9. LUESSENHOP, A. J., KACHMANN, R., SHEVLIN, W., FERRERO, A. A.: Clinical evaluation of artefical embolisation in the management of large cerebral arteriovenous malformations. J. Neurosurg. 23, 400-417 (1965).

10. PAMPUS, F., TZONOS, T., BERGLEITER, R.: Treatment of angiomas and aneurysmas without direct surgical attack. J. Neurosurg. Sci. (Milano) 17, 18-22 (1973).

11. ROBLES, C., CARRASCO-ZANINI, J.: Treatment of cerebral arteriovenous malformations by muscle embolisation. J. Neurosurg. 29, 603-608 (1968).

12. ROSENBLUTH, P. R., GROSSMAN, R., ARIAS, B.: Accurate placement of artificial emboli. J. Amer. med. Ass. 174, 308-309 (1960).

13. TZONOS, T., BERGLEITER, R.: Behandlung von inoperablen Hirnangiomen durch artefizielle Embolisierung. Z. Neurol. 200, 45-50 (1971).

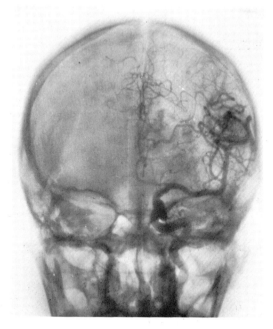

Fig. 1. Carotid arteriogram in antero-posterior view showing a considerable hypertrophy of the left middle cerebral trunk and a faint staining of pathological vessels projecting towards the Sylvian fissure

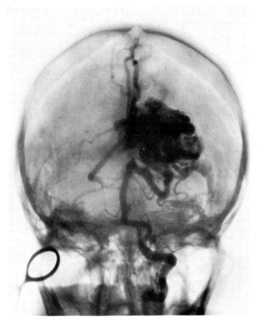

Fig. 2. An antero-posterior view of the left vertebral artery showing the enlarged feeding vessels of the malformation extending up to the midline from the posterior cerebral artery

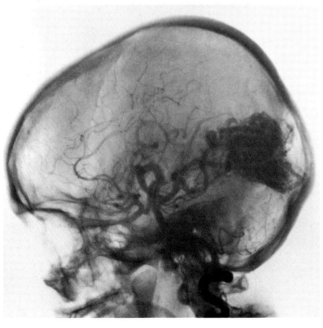

Fig. 3. A lateral vertebral arteriogram with compression of the left internal carotid localizing the malformation in the occipital region with feeding branches also from the posterior inferior cerebellar artery

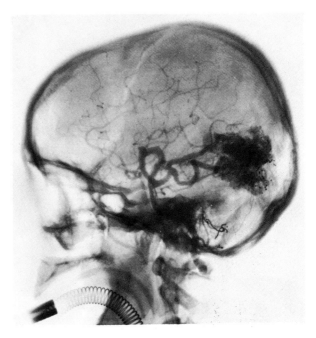

Fig. 4. Lateral view of the vertebral angiogram with compression of the left internal carotid after embolization with 1 mm emboli, introduced percutaneously via the femoral artery. Apparent reduction of the malformation. There are many emboli in the posterior inferior cerebellar artery. Decrease in size of the branch of the middle cerebral artery

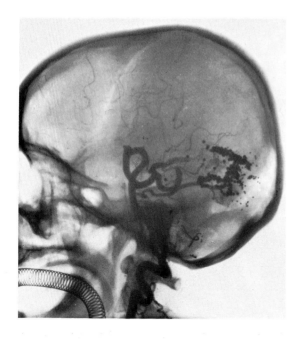

Fig. 5

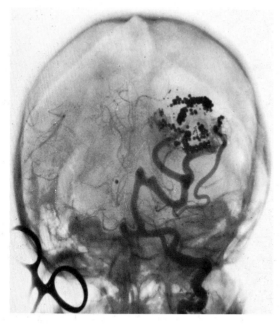

Fig. 6

Figs. 5 and 6. Final stage demonstrated by vertebral arteriogram after embolization with appr. 170 emboli from 2 to 2.5 mm diameter, directly introduced into the vertebral artery. These emboli occlude almost completely the malformation. One aberrant embolus passed into the right posterior cerebral artery without producing abnormal clinical findings

The Artificial Embolization of Inoperable Angiomas

W. SEEGER

Previous reports have discussed the method* used in artificial embolization. The following points arise from our initial experiences of this
technique:

first: the problems of the indication for embolization
second: the problems of the technique of artificial embolization
third: the problems of the interpretation of the results.

The first problem is the indication for embolization. The brain stem
is not the exclusive site for the location of an inoperable angioma.
They have a preference for the dominant hemisphere and its parietal region. The problems of this kind of angioma are different from brain
stem angiomas but by no means less difficult. Their total elimination
by artificial embolization or a partial occlusion combined with subsequent operative extirpation of the remnants is desirable, but often
it is not possible or not indicated because of the risks involved. The
discovery on angiography of an unfavourable course of the feeding vessels is a limiting factor in the indication for embolization, as you
have heard in the proceeding reports. In most cases of inoperable angiomas artificial embolization will produce only partial elimination of
the malformation. The findings and the results in this group of partially eliminated angiomas provide important information in forming a
criterion for the indication and prognosis of artificial embolization.

It is well known that angiomas enlarge again after an incomplete operative extirpation (TÖNNIS). How quickly this is possible after artificial embolization, the following case demonstrates.

There is seen an angioma originating from big branches of the middle
cerebral artery in the parietal region of the dominant hemisphere. The
angioma is visible medially and is also supplied by a small branch from
the anterior cerebral artery (Fig. 1). The clinical picture of tetraparesis indicated that the cerebral circulation was generally decreased.
Angiographic studies of the vertebro-basilar circulation showed no angioma in the brain stem or upper spinal cord.

After embolization of the biggest of the feeding vessels, the branches
of the middle cerebral artery became smaller, as expected, but after a
few weeks, repeated angiography revealed an enlargement of the anterior
cerebral artery and the small feeding vessels between the anterior cerebral artery and the angioma.

---

* method of Luessenhop

Embolization of these vessels was impossible because the bifurcation of the carotid artery showed a normal configuration with the anterior cerebral artery leaving the bifurcation at an acute angle. It can be seen, however, that the cerebral circulation was improved (Fig. 2).

The angioma showed slow filling with contrast medium and was smaller than before, being visualized in the early venous phase of the angiogram. The clinical result was ambivalent also. The same severe neurological deficits were found before and after embolization (Fig. 3).

The second case illustrates the problem of the difficulties in operative technique. It was an angioma of the middle cerebral artery in the dominant hemisphere. The patient suffered from focal epilepsy. 13 years previously a subdural hematoma had been evacuated without complications. At first, we tried to close the arteriovenous fistulae with small emboli (Fig. 4). Check X-ray showed, however, that the emboli having passed the arteriovenous fistulae had reached the arteries of the lungs. We then used bigger emboli of diameter from 1.5 to 2.0 and 2.5 mm. This small difference in size brought about complete occlusion of both the big branches of the middle cerebral artery. One of these two branches disappeared totally on the angiogram; the other can be seen, filled indirectly through collaterals.

In this postoperative angiogram slow filling of the angioma in the venous phase occurred together with enlargement of the anterior cerebral artery. On the clinical side there has been no further epilepsy but the follow-up period is only 8 months (Fig. 5).

In addition to these two cases we have seen 2 similar cases with angiomata of the middle cerebral territory in the dominant hemisphere, one of which showed an intermittently progressive hemiparesis after embolization. These experiences lead on to the third point of interest, i.e. the interpretation of the operative results. The first case showed significant improvement in the immediate postoperative angiogram without clinical benefit and with an early recurrence. The second example showed occlusion of the middle cerebral artery after artificial embolization without elimination of the angioma, though clinically the epilepsy was abolished and there were no neurological deficits. Then there remains a question as to which factors determine the operative results.

In all cases partial or total filling of the angioma was seen after embolization in the early venous phase, and the circulation time in the malformation was consistently slower than before embolization. Serial angiography must be done in order to show all phases of the circulation. Control angiography is able to show the early recurrence of the angioma.

S u m m a r y

Particular technical requirements limit the indications for embolization of inoperable angiomas. The dominating problem is the recurrence or enlargement of only incompletely occluded malformations. Paradoxical effects are possible i.e. improvement in the angiographic picture without clinical benefit or per contra failure of embolization of the angioma though there was occlusion of the middle cerebral artery branches followed by an improvement in the clinical picture.

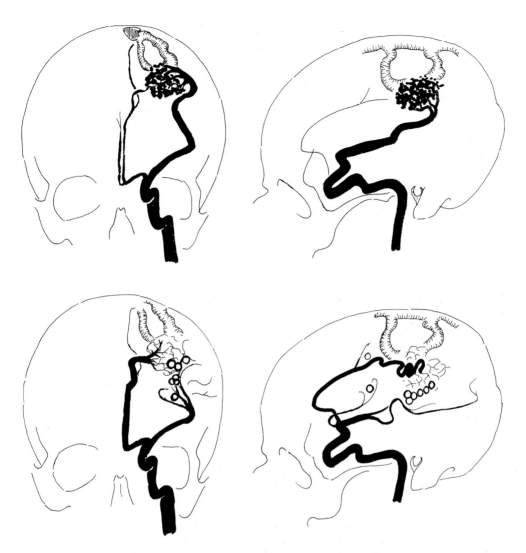

Fig. 1. Preoperative angiogram. The angioma is fed by major cerebral arteries.
Below: Four weeks after embolization the angioma is smaller. Enlargement of the anterior cerebral artery and feeding of the angioma by an enlarged branch between the anterior cerebral artery and the angioma

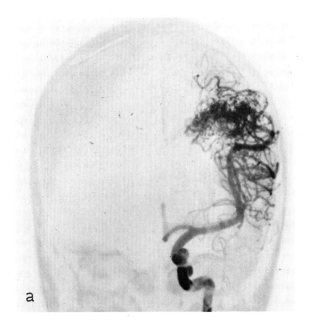

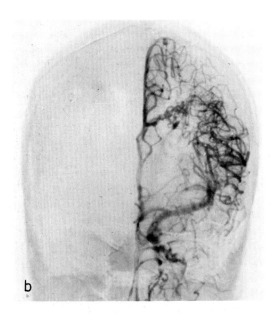

Fig. 2 a and b. Original angioma of the same case

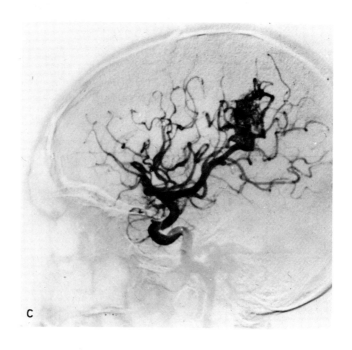

c

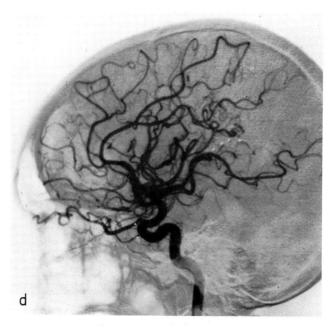

d

Fig. 2 c and d. Original angioma of the same case

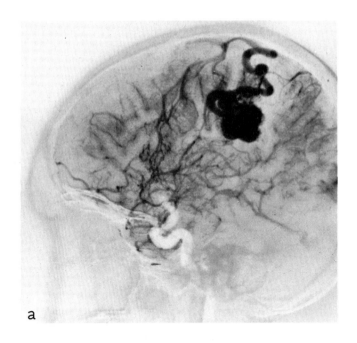

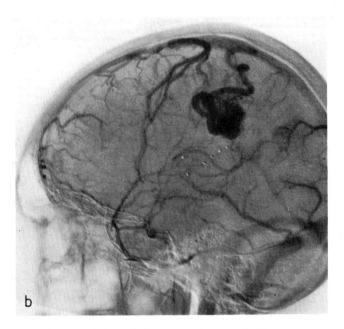

Fig. 3 a and b. a) Venous phase of the angiogram preoperatively.
b) Only in the venous phase can the angioma be seen after embolization.
It has decreased in size

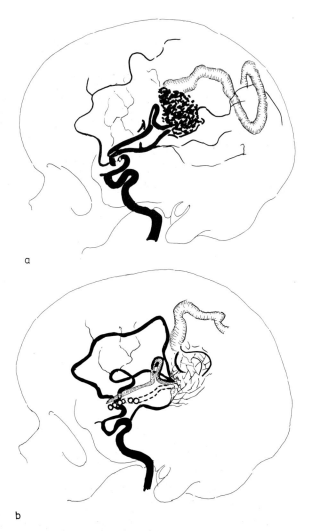

a

b

Fig. 4 a and b. a) AVM fed by big branches of the middle cerebral artery. b) Both feeding arteries have been closed by embolization of the trunk of the middle cerebral artery. Retrograde filling of the upper feeding artery

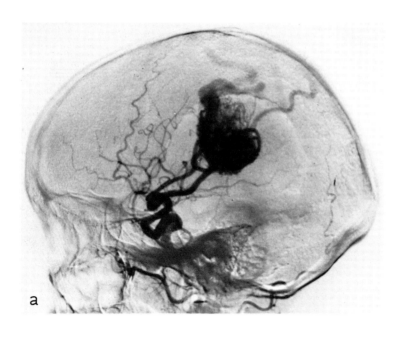

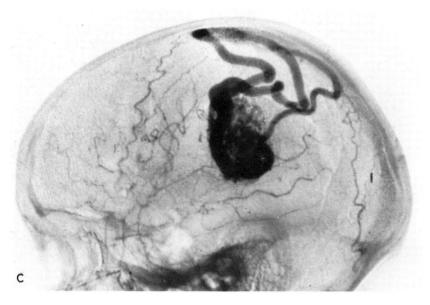

Fig. 5 a - d. Angiogram of the same case as in Fig. 4. a and c pre-operative angiogram, b and d postoperative angiogram

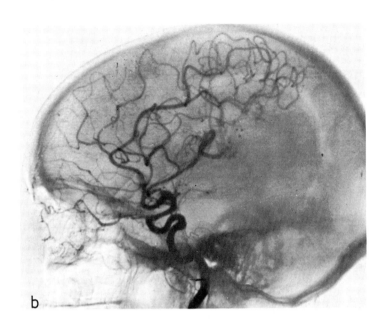

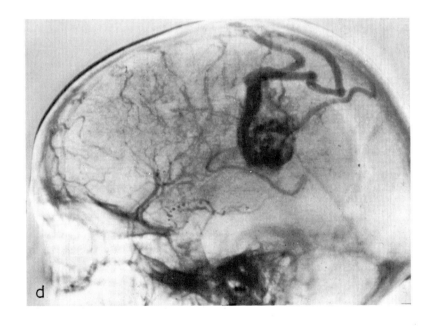

Artificial Embolization of Inoperable Angioma with Polymerizing Substance

K. Sano, M. Jimbo, I. Saito and N. Basugi

Introduction

Of 205 cases of arteriovenous malformations (angiomas) of the brain which have been seen at the Department of Neurosurgery, University of Tokyo, 192 cases have been followed up for a period from one to 24 years.

As seen in Table 1, 37 per cent of the cases which were treated non-surgically (i.e. conservatively) eventually died mostly from hemorrhage or recurrent hemorrhage. This high mortality was particularly notice-able in the deep-seated arteriovenous malformations which had a 50 per cent mortality and in the very large ones which showed a 33 per cent mortality.

Table 1. Follow-up of AVM (1-24 years) - Results (192 cases). For fur-ther explanation see text

Surgically treated cases		Excellent	Good	Fair	Poor	Died
Cortical	107	44	47	5	2	9
Deep-seated	30	8	12	4	1	5
Very large	20	1	3	8	2	6
Infratentorial	8	5	1	0	0	2
Total	165	58	63	17	5	22 %
	(100)	(35.2)	(38.2)	(10.3)	(3.0)	(13.3)

Non-surgically treated cases						
Cortical	5	0	4	1	0	0
Deep-seated	14	3	4	0	0	7
Very large	6	1	3	0	0	2
Infratentorial	2	1	0	0	0	1
Total	27	5	11	1	0	10 %
	(100)	(18.5)	(40.8)	(3.7)		(37.0)

An arteriovenous malformation (AVM) consists of the feeding arteries, the draining vessels and the anomalous arteriovenous shunts (the nidus). In this Table "cortical" means that the nidus was located near the cortical surface and its diameter was less than 3 cm. If the nidus was located in the paraventricular area, the basal ganglia or the brain stem, the malformation is designated as "deep-seated". If the nidus was more than 4 or 5 cm in diameter and occupying more than one cerebral lobe or a whole hemisphere, the malformation is called "very large".

In contrast to the non-surgical cases, 165 cases were treated by surgery and showed a mortality of 13.3 per cent, namely about one third of that of the former group in the follow-up (22 cases which included 8 cases of postoperative hospital death i.e. 4.7 per cent). These deaths were due to epileptic seizures or recurrent hemorrhage resulting from incomplete extirpation of the AVM. Not only the mortality, but also the morbidity, was lower in the surgical cases than in the non-surgical cases. In Table 1, "excellent" means that the cases have no neurological deficit, no recurrent hemorrhage, no epileptic seizures, and are leading a useful life. "Good" means that the cases may have some kind or degree of neurological deficit or epileptic seizures, although they are leading a useful life. By "fair" it is meant that the cases can take care of themselves, although they are unable to work for society. "Poor" means that the cases are bedridden. In the surgically treated cases, the "excellent" group was 35.2 per cent and the "good" group was 38.2 per cent, figures which are better than for the comparable groups in the non-surgical cases.

These data suggest that one should try to extirpate AVM wherever possible. This is true even with the paraventricular AVM. Table 2 shows a recent series of 10 cases with these malformations. In 4 cases neurological deficits which were not present before the operation appeared postoperatively, but they are all leading useful lives.

Table 2. Paraventricular AVM

case	age	Location	Hematoma	Pre-op	Post-op	op
1	35M	lt-central	+	hemiplegia	→	extirpation
2	20M	rt-frontal	+	hemiparesis	→	extirpation
3	25M	lt-central	+	n. p.	hemiparesis	extirpation
4	15F	lt-central	+	n. p.	n. p.	extirpation
5	17F	lt-central	+	n. p.	n. p.	extirpation
6	40M	rt-thalamus	+	hemiplegia	→	extirpation
7	12F	rt-thalamus	-	n. p.	hemianopia	extirpation
8	27M	rt-central	-	n. p.	n. p.	extirpation
9	21M	rt-thalamus	-	D. T. R.↑	hemiplegia	clipping
10	27M	rt-thalamus	-	n. p.	hemiparesis	extirpation

M: male, F: female, Hematoma: accompanying intracerebral hematoma, n. p.: no neurological deficit. D. T. R. : increased deep reflex, D. T. R.: the same as the preoperative status.

The problem is "the very large" AVM which can not be extirpated without causing neurological deficits. For the treatment of this kind of AVM, the authors have been performing artificial embolization.

First the authors tried to inject spherical emboli, as reported by LUESSENHOP (2, 3). The spherical emboli consisted of a radiopaque barium sulphate ball covered with silicon rubber and were from 2.3 mm to 4.5 mm in diameter, the specific gravity being 3.0. The emboli were injected one by one into the internal carotid through a catheter inserted into the external carotid artery under X-ray control (image intensifier and angiography) and observing closely the neurological signs and symptoms (6).

13 cases of AVM underwent this procedure as summarized in the upper half of Table 3. Main feeding arteries were from the M_1 portion of the middle cerebral artery (4 cases), from the M_2, and M_3 segments (2 cases), from the M_4 segment (5 cases), from the posterior cerebral artery (one case), and from the anterior cerebral artery (one case). (The nomenclature M_{1-4} is according to FISCHER (1)). Emboli used varied from 5 to 66 in number.

Table 3. Artificial embolization with spherical emboli and liquid plastics. Follow up (5-10 years) - operative results

method	main feed.a.	cases	nidus(-) defi-cit(-)	nidus(-) defi-cit(+)	nidus(+) defi-cit(-)	nidus(+) defi-cit(+)	died
Spheric. Emboli	M1	4	1		1	2	
	M2, 3	2		1			1
	M4	5			3	2	
	others	2				1	1
	Total	13	1	1	4	5	2
Liquid Plastic	M1	0					
	M2, 3	3		1	1	1	
	M4	4	1	1	2		
	others	1			1		
	Total	8	1	2	4	1	0
Total		21	2	3	8	6	2

nidus (-): nidus not demonstrated in angiogram, deficit (-): no neurological deficit, (+): reverse.

As seen in Table 3, the AVM (nidus) became obliterated or almost obliterated angiographically in 2 cases. Neurological deficits were not encountered in 5 cases and found in 6. There was no case of rebleeding after the procedure. The follow up was from 6 to 10 years.

The fact that there was no rebleeding after embolization, even though the AVM could still be demonstrated by angiography, may be explained by the supposition that the blood volume or pressure in the nidus has been decreased by this procedure. There were, however, two cases of postoperative death due to brain edema caused by embolization of main arterial branches. This experience led the authors to use a liquid plastic rather than spherical emboli (7).

Furthermore, the direction of flow of emboli seems more dependent on the anatomical course of the feeding arteries rather than their contained blood volume, so that spherical emboli tend to lodge in one feeding artery like a string of beads and consequently the nidus of AVM remains and is supplied by other feeding arteries (Fig. 1 and Fig. 2 right upper). The middle cerebral artery is the anatomical continuation of the internal carotid artery. Artificial embolization is indicated when the feeding (afferent) arteries of the AVM are the anatomical continuation of the middle cerebral artery which is itself the physiological feeding artery (5) (Fig. 3 A). Thus a very large AVM in the region of M_4 is a good candidate for the artificial embolization.

If the feeders come off the main stem at a right-angle or obtuse angle as in Fig. 3 B, this procedure is not indicated. Therefore embolization of AVM fed by the anterior cerebral or posterior cerebral arteries is contraindicated.

When the nidus is located in the region of M_1, M_2 or M_3, artificial embolization may be dangerous because the main trunk of the middle cerebral artery may be embolized (Fig. 3 C). One of the 2 cases of postoperative death after the procedure had an AVM in the region of M_2 and the other case had an AVM in the region of the posterior cerebral artery.

A r t i f i c i a l   E m b o l i z a t i o n   w i t h   L i q u i d
P l a s t i c

As mentioned above, spherical emboli do not enter the plexiform nidus of an AVM and therefore the nidus remains to be supplied by many feeding arteries other than the embolized one (Fig. 2 right upper). If a liquid plastic which could enter the plexiform nidus, lodge there, and polymerize there were available, it would be an ideal embolizing substance.

Phycon 6500 seems to be such a substance. This is a liquid silicone rubber (dimethyl polysiloxane), the specific gravity being 0.98 (at 25° C) and its viscosity being 10,000 centi-poise (at 25° C). When one drop of the catalyst HL is added to 5 ml of Phycon, polymeriaztion begins in about 1 1/2 minutes and is completed in about 3 minutes. It becomes a rubber-like elastic substance and no heat is produced.

The Phycon can enter the nidus of an AVM, but can not pass into the draining vessels because of its viscosity. It therefore remains in the network of the nidus to polymerize there (Fig. 2 right lower).

After adding the catalyst, the liquid plastic was injected in aliquots into the internal carotid artery through a catheter in the external carotid, the volume of each injection being 0.2 - 0.5 ml, under X-ray control (image intensifier and angiography). The total volume injected was between 2 ml and 24.4 ml. There were 8 cases treated by this procedure (Table 3 lower half). There was no postoperative death. In the follow up lasting from 5 to 8 years, there was no case of bleeding or rebleeding. The nidus was obliterated on the angiogram in 3 cases and decreased in size in 5 cases. There were 5 cases without neurological deficits and 3 cases with neurological deficits postoperatively.

Fig. 4 a, b are the angiograms of a 17-year-old girl who had repeated attacks of generalized convulsions and a left hemiparesis. Fig. 5 a, b are the angiograms after injection of 5.7 ml of Phycon and clipping of the right anterior cerebral artery. The AVM is only faintly demonstrated, and this is the portion supplied by the anterior cerebral artery; the portion fed by the middle cerebral artery has been obliterated by Phycon.

The indication for Phycon injection is the same as for embolization with spherical emboli. Phycon injection, however, seems much better than the latter in the sense that the liquid plastic enters and stays in the plexiform nidus of the AVM. There have never been any signs of toxicity of this substance.

As reported previously (4), the authors have performed a quantitative measurement of intracerebral arteriovenous shunt flow by means of cerebro-pulmonary scanning using I-131 labeled macroaggregated human serum albumin (MAA). The relative shunt flow, namely the radioactivity of the lungs divided by the radioactivity of the skull plus the radioactivity of the lungs after intracarotid injection of I-131 MAA shows values of 5.73 to 10.73 in the normal control, whereas it is 26.0 to 76.75 in cases with AVM. When extirpation or embolization of the AVM was complete, the measurement of the relative shunt flow showed normal values. This method may be an adjunct to angiography in the assessment of the results of surgery of AVM.

R e f e r e n c e s

1. FISCHER, E.: Die Lageabweichungen der vorderen Hirnarterie im Gefässbild. Zbl. Neurochir., 3, 300-313 (1938).

2. LUESSENHOP, A. J., SPENCE, W. T.: Artificial embolization of cerebral arteries. Report of use in a case of arteriovenous malformation. J. A. M. A. 172, 1153-1155 (1960).

3. LUESSENHOP, A. J., KACHMANN, R. Jr., SHEVLIN, W., FERRERO, A. A.: Clinical evaluation of artificial embolization in the management of large cerebral arteriovenous malformations. J. Neurosurg., 23, 400-417 (1965).

4. NAGAI, T., JIMBO, M., SANO, K.: Cerebro-pulmonary scan using macroaggregated albumin as a quantitation of intracerebral arteriovenous shunting. J. Nucl. Med., 8, 709-722 (1967).

5. OLIVECRONA, H., LADENHEIM, J.: Congenital arteriovenous aneurysms of the carotid and vertebral arterial systems. Berlin: Springer 1957.

6. SANO, K.: Intracranial arteriovenous malformation with special reference to its treatment. Neurol. med.-chir., 6, 28-34 (1964).

7. SANO, K., JIMBO, M., SAITO, I., TERAO, H., HIRAKAWA, K.: Artificial embolization with liquid plastic. Neurol. med.-chir., 8, 198-201 (1966).

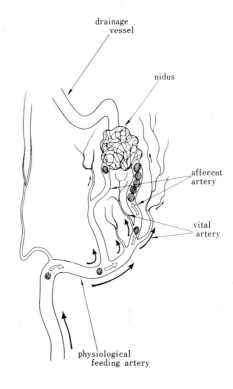

Fig. 1

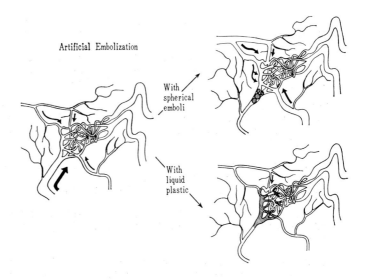

Fig. 2

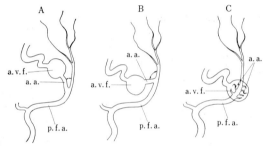

a.a. : afferent artery
p.f.a. : physiological feeding artery
a.v.f. : arterio-venous fistula

Fig. 3

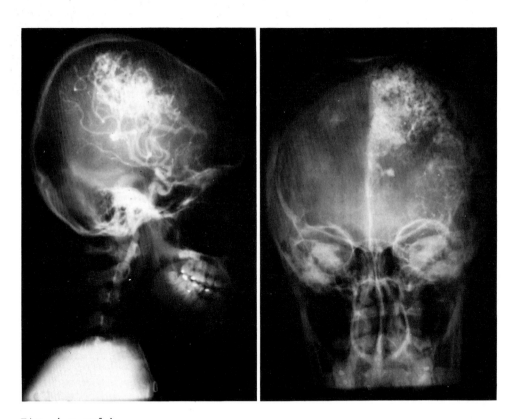

Fig. 4 a and b

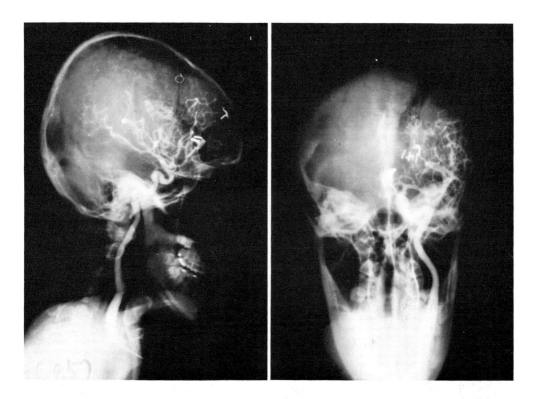

Fig. 5 a and b

Extra-Cerebral Embolization

R. DJINDJIAN

The embolization of inoperable cerebral arteriovenous malformations
was introduced by LUESSENHOP who embolized these malformations from
the extra-cranial carotid artery using silastic spheroids. Numerous
authors have since used this method, modifying either the nature of
the emboli (china beads, metallic beads, fragments of muscle, gelfoam)
or extending the indications for embolization to include cerebral angiomas, dural malformations supplied by the external carotid artery
and vertebral angiomas.

All the authors have carried out cerebral embolization by a cervical
approach: either introducing the emboli by a percutaneous catheter into the common carotid artery, or retrogradely via the external carotid artery following surgical exposure, or lastly into the internal carotid itself. Whatever the nature of the emboli, then usually follow
the increased blood-flow supplying the malformation, and Luessenhop
has shown that silastic beads may take 24 hours or more to reach their
ultimate destination. In some cases, the beads may not reach the malformation and may lodge in normal arteries. One case has been reported
of beads having obstructed the ophthalmic artery, thus causing blind-
ness, in another case, the beads migrated into the lungs, but without
any pathological signs.

The advent of super-selective angiographic technique such as we have
been performing for about 3 years permits the precise visualization
of the malformation: the different feeders and the main supplying vessels. This technique suggested a new application of embolization to us
and we have applied it to numerous extra-cerebral diseases.

Aim of Embolization

The aim of embolization may be considered under different headings.
If surgical intervention is not possible because of the site or the
morphology of the malformation, or on account of the clinical state
of the patient, embolization seems capable of obliterating the malformation or at least reducing its volume. Of course, this may not totally prevent a hemorrhage, but it enables one to diminish the "steal"
resulting from the arteriovenous fistula and consequently to improve
the vascularisation of the neighboring parenchyma.

Lastly embolization does not preclude surgical intervention. In a few
cerebral or medullary tumors, it may be considered as a step prepara-

230

tory to surgery, either to reduce the risk of hemorrhage by diminishing the blood-flow, or to do away with certain inoperable or difficult
feeding vessels and consequently to reduce the number of operations.

P e r s o n a l   T e c h n i q u e   o f   E m b o l i z a t i o n

1. Our technique of embolization is based on two principles which at
first may seem contradictory. The emboli must be injected in a superselective way after catheterisation of the pathological vessel which
necessitates the use of a tapered tip, and yet the emboli must have
sufficient volume to obstruct the pathological vessel.

2. The use of the femoral approach for introducing a catheter with a
tapered tip enables one to enter the terminal branches of the external carotid artery i.e. the internal maxillary, superficial temporal,
middle meningeal, occipital, lingual, and facial arteries. The femoro-
cerebral approach is far less traumatic than the puncture and cannula-
tion of the cervical carotid artery which may cause spasm of the artery or establish a site for thrombosis and embolization.

3. The use of a catheter with a tapered tip precludes embolization with
silastic beads which are too big to pass out of the catheter. One must
choose either muscle or gelfoam and we have now discarded the former
in favour of the latter. Gelfoam has the advantage of not requiring
surgery to obtain it: it is more malleable than muscle and passes more
easily through the catheter. It is easily cut into fine strips about
one centimeter long and repeated emboli are easily injected into the
feeding artery under TV control.

4. Embolization with gelfoam, muscle, or silastic can not be compared
with arterial ligature. The aim of embolization is to induce natural
thrombosis by means of a foreign substance (a substance which is readily absorbed). The natural thrombosis proceeds to occlude the arteries
in a more permanent manner and perhaps propagates sufficiently actually
to occlude the fistula itself (KRICHEFF).

5. After embolization it is necessary to perform serial angiography to
assess the result: one must not be satisfied with a single film. During the following months we perform control arteriography which enables
one to judge the effectiveness of the thrombosis on the pathological
feeders. If necessary the embolization of new feeders which may have
appeared later can be carried out.

L i m i t s   a n d   D a n g e r s   o f   E m b o l i z a t i o n

1. The quantity of contrast material injected is necessarily of importance because of the multiplicity of injections needed in spite of the
introduction of the catheter into the external carotid artery.

2. It is necessary to carry out precise selective catheterisation of
the branches of the external carotid artery because of the risk of
back-flow of emboli into the common carotid artery and then into the
internal carotid artery.

Superselective catheterisation of the branches of the external carotid
artery is not always easy. The internal maxillary artery and middle

meningeal artery sometimes have curves that prevent the introduction of the catheter.

3. Embolization of the feeders of a malformation causes a dilatation of the neighboring arteries and one may occasionally see muscle branches filling abnormally from adjacent vessels. In some cases it is necessary to embolize these arteries because they are part of the blood supply of the malformation.

P a t h o l o g i c a l   C a s e s

The external carotid territory provides an ideal situation for embolization because of the possibility of super-selectivity on the one hand and the absence of the risk of cerebral ischemia on the other.

a) In <u>vascular malformations</u> supplied by one or several branches of the external carotid artery, embolization seems the most satisfactory method.

Dural angiomas in the posterior fossa (Figs. 1, 2, 3) seem to be the most frequent form of abnormality and can easily be embolized because the main feeding vessel is the dilated occipital artery. Sometimes both occipital arteries take part in the blood supply of the malformation. In certain cases, the participation of feeders from other territories is found e.g. the meningeal artery of the tent (a branch of the internal carotid artery) and the posterior meningeal artery arising from the vertebral artery and here there is no possibility of embolization of course.

Other malformations are filled from the middle meningeal artery (Figs. 4, 5) or from the posterior auricular and ascending pharyngeal arteries.

It is necessary before embolization of these dural malformations to carry out complete selective arteriography of all the posterior branches of the external carotid artery together with the internal carotid, the vertebral, the ascending and deep cervical arteries, and also the other side.

Carotid angiography permits the discovery of new feeding vessels and allows fresh embolization if necessary.

b) <u>Angiomas fed by the anterior branches of the external carotid artery.</u>

Examples are:

1. An angioma of the forehead filled by the right and left superficial temporal arteries (Fig. 6).

2. A nasal angioma filled from the facial artery (and its tributaries especially the nasal artery), from the internal maxillary artery by the infra-orbital artery and its terminal branches, and from the spheno-palatine artery. Embolization of the facial artery may be carried out in certain cases of catastrophic epistaxis (Fig. 7).

3. An angiolipoma of the face fed by the facial artery (Figs. 8, 9).

4. An angioma of the tongue opacified from the lingual artery (Fig. 10). Some authors recommend the embolization of the lingual artery before

difficult teeth extractions or in angiomata of the maxillary bone to prevent catastrophic hemorrhage from the gums.

Conclusions

Our conclusions are:

1. Embolization is now the best emergency treatment for epistaxis and dental and lingual hemorrhage.

2. In small dural malformations with one or several feeding vessels, embolization give good results.

3. In big dural malformations with many feeders, embolization may be considered where:

a) surgical ligation of the several feeding vessels would necessitate many operations.

b) resection of the malformation is dangerous. In such cases pre-operative embolization seems the best technique.

4. Embolization and surgery seem a good combination in certain cases. We use this technique in the Lariboisiere hospital in all tumors fed by the external carotid artery: metastases (Fig. 11), naso-pharyngeal angio-fibromata, glomic tumors, and especially meningiomata pre-operatively. This technique avoids the risk of catastrophic hemorrhage during operation and it is a very big step forward in neuroradiology and neurosurgery.

References

DJINDJIAN, R., et al.: Neuroradiology, Vol. 6, 1, 20-26 (1973).

DJINDJIAN, R., et al.: Neuroradiology, Vol. 6, 3, 132-142 (1973).

DJINDJIAN, R., et al.: Neuroradiology, Vol. 6, 3, 143-153 (1973).

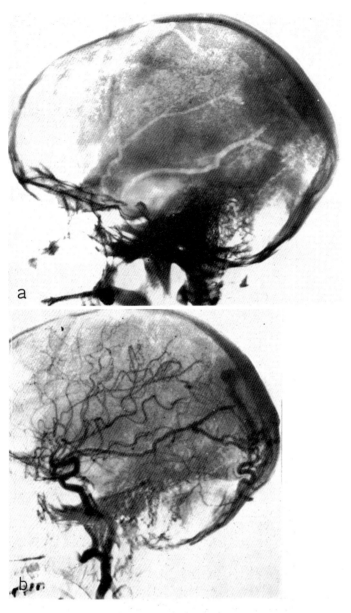

Fig. 1 a. Vascular malformations of the skull and dura of the posterior fossa. Vascular channels on the lateral plain film

Fig. 1 b. Common carotid angiography: opacification of the occipital
malformation

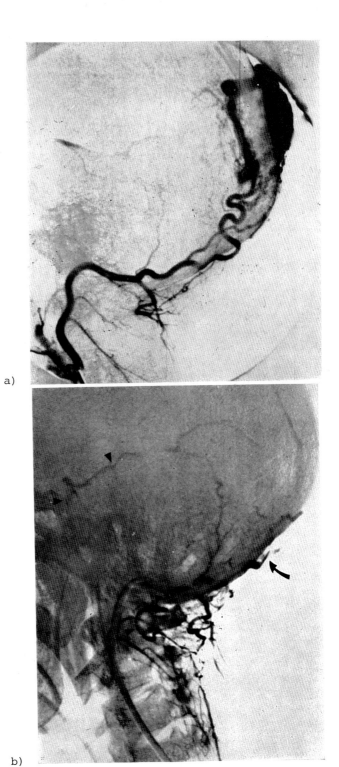

a)

b)

Fig. 2 a and b.
a) Same case: selective angiography of the occipital artery. b) After embolization

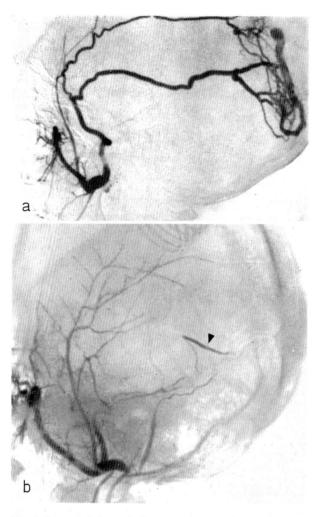

Fig. 3 a and b. a) Same case: selective arteriography of the middle
meningeal artery. b) after embolization

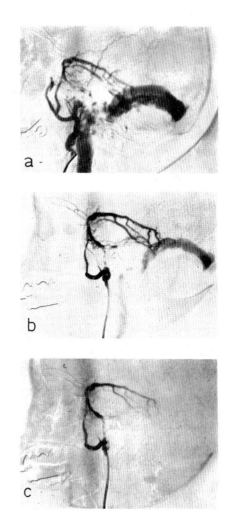

Fig. 4. Dural fistula between the middle meningeal artery and the lateral sinus. a) Selective arteriography of the terminal branches of the external carotid artery. b) Super-selective arteriography of the middle meningeal artery (late phase). c) Early phase

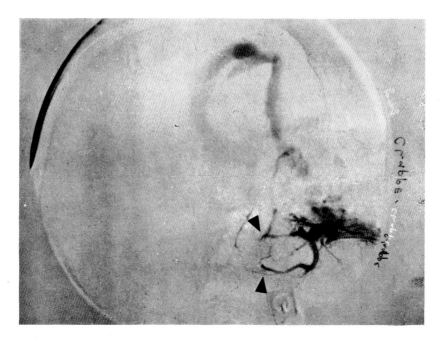

Fig. 5. Same case after embolization

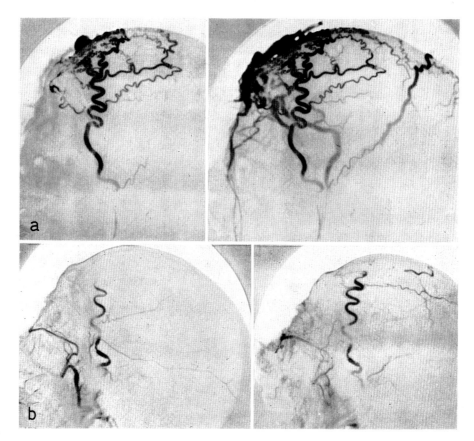

Fig. 6 a and b. Vascular malformations of forehead.
a) Superselective angiography of the feeding vessel, the anterior branch of the superficial temporal artery (early and late phases).
b) After embolization (early and late pahses)

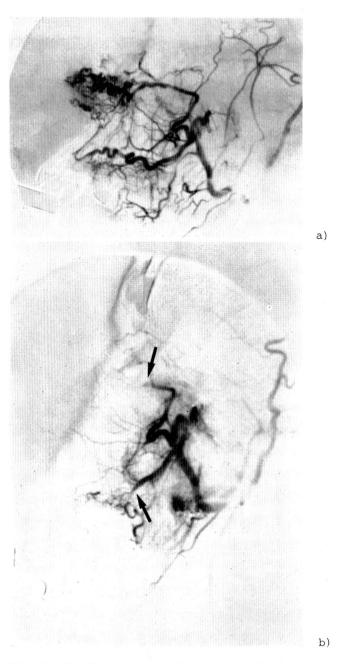

a)

b)

Fig. 7. Nasal angioma with catastrophic epistaxis.
a) Super-selective arteriography of the internal maxillary artery.
b) After embolization

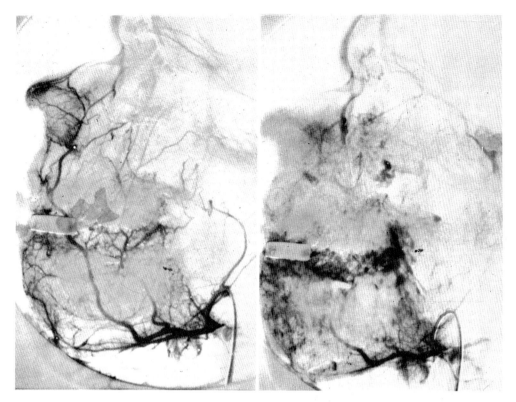

Fig. 8. Massive facial angioma and lymphangioma. a and b. Superselective arteriography of the facial artery (early and late phase)

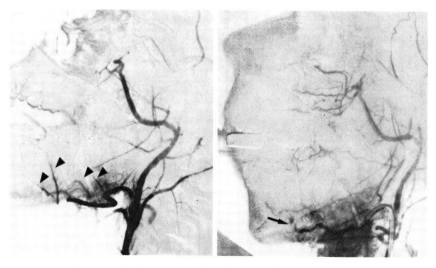

Fig. 9. Same case after embolization (early and late phase)

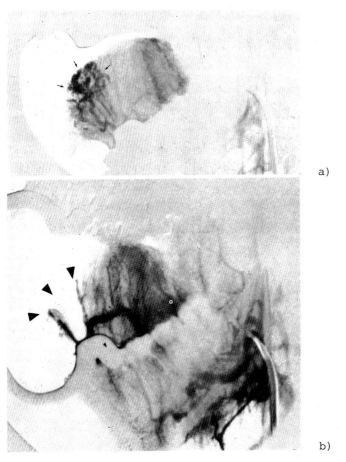

a)

b)

Fig. 10 a and b. Lingual angioma. a) Super-selective arteriography of
the lingual artery. b) After embolization

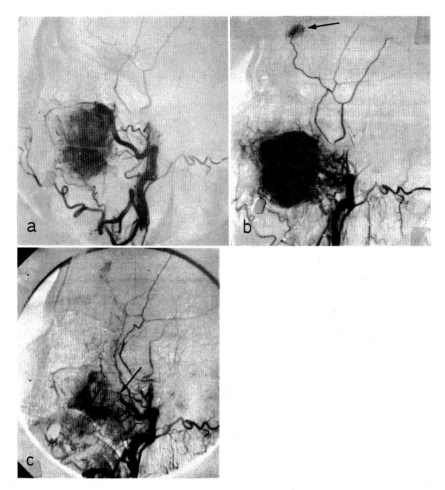

Fig. 11 a - c. Metastatic lesion of the maxillary sinus. a and b)
Super-selective arteriography of the internal maxillary artery.
c) After embolization

Treatment of Inoperable Glomus Jugulare Tumors

R. E. M. HEKSTER

In our hospital we have been using the transcatheter embolization technique in the treatment of large glomus jugulare tumors expanding into the petrous temporal bone. Up to the present only patients for whom no other treatment was considered acceptable have been selected for transcatheter occlusion therapy.

Because glomus jugulare tumors (chemodectoma) are uncommon our experience is limited. We feel however, that occlusion by embolization of the feeding vessels of these very vascular tumors, a technique including thrombosis in the zones supplied, has definite advantages compared with operation and radiotherapy. In our view the method represents in large glomus tumors, which are considered inoperable by normal standards, a practical alternative to other methods of treatment. The method seems to be extremely useful in controlling, at least temporarily, the expansion of the lesion. The treatment can be repeated if necessary.

Since 1971 five patients with inoperable glomus jugulare tumors have been treated with occlusion by transcatheter embolization of the feeding vessels by our team (headed by professor W. LUYENDIJK).

Muscle from the patient's thigh has been selected as being the most suitable material for therapeutic embolization, gelfoam is used for presurgical embolization purposes. Thin radiopaque catheters inserted via the femoral artery are used. The tumor feeding vessels previously identified during diagnostic angiography are selectively catheterized and muscle (or gelfoam) strips measuring approximately 2x2x 4-10 mm are then introduced into the catheter and injected mannually into the artery by means of a follow-through injection of diluted contrast medium.

In our patients no further progression of the neurological deficit or clinical symptomatology necessitating some form of treatment was noted after embolization. All 5 patients showed definite clinical improvement.

One patient with a very large tumor which had been considered inoperable due to its size and location was repeatedly treated by embolization until, 32 months and four procedures after initial treatment, she underwent operation. Complete removal of the tumor was achieved. The patient was discharged in excellent condition a month after operation. Figs. 1, 2 demonstrate the size of this patient's lesion.

In the material removed at operation large areas of thrombosed and necrotic tumor tissue were found. An inflammatory reaction of the vessel wall with adherent embolus-material from the last, presurgical embolization, is demonstrated (Fig. 3). (dr. G. TH. A. M. BOTS, neuropathologist).

References

HEKSTER, R. E. M., LUYENDIJK, W., MATRICALI, B.: Transfemoral catheter embolization: a method of treatment of glomus jugulare tumors. Neuroradiology, 5, 208-214 (1973)

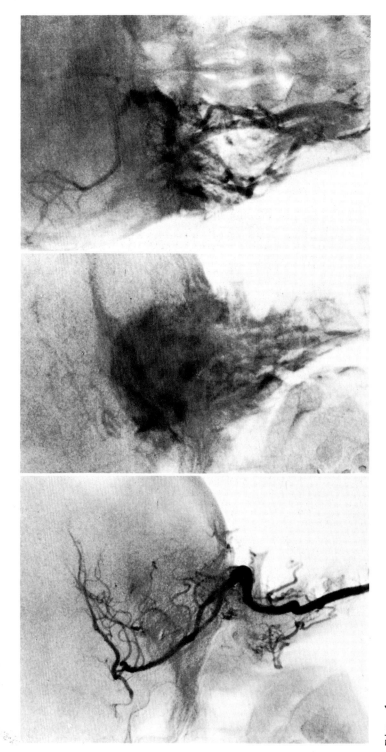

Fig. 1

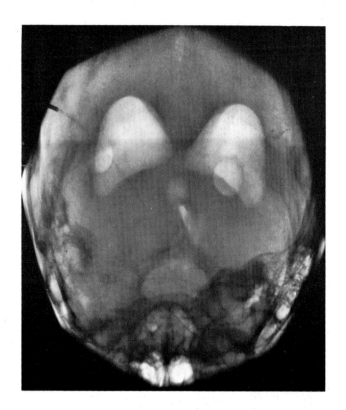

Fig. 2

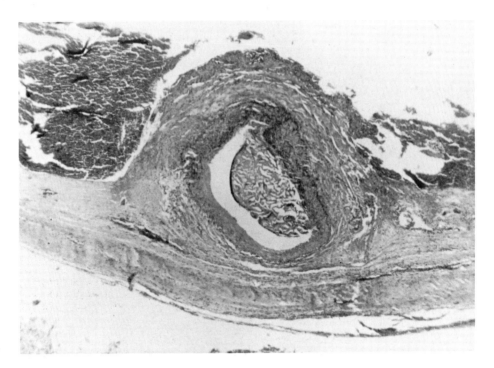

Fig. 3 a

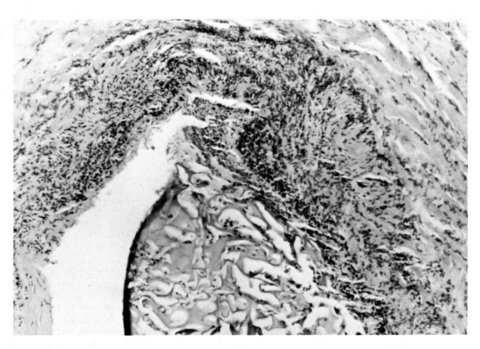

Fig. 3 b

Discussion on Chapter VII

PIA: Embolization for the treatment of carotico-cavernous fistulas was introduced in 1930 by BROOKS. The procedure remained limited in scope because of unpredictable risks. It was Dr. Luessenhop who in 1962 took the decisive step of embolizing of inoperable a-v angiomas. He completed the procedure and combined it with primary or secondary extirpation. Being effective, it opened a new area of treatment and was accepted and modified by many authors

HEMMER: Artificial embolization of an arteriovenous aneurysm (sinus cavernosus) of the right internal carotid artery and basilar artery.

We are dealing with a 9-year-old boy who entered the hospital after a traffic accident with a cerebral concussion and fracture of the lower jaw. After 3 weeks he showed an increasing right-sided exophthalmus with a pulssynchronous murmur, predominantly over the frontal region. Other than double images when looking to the right and upward, there were no pathological findings neurologically. The angiogram showed an aneurysm about the size of a cherry, which was fed by the right internal carotid artery as well as by the basilar artery. In addition, there was a typical enlargement of the ophthalmic vein. We planned at first to conduct the embolization using means of silastic balls (spence spheres) starting from the internal carotid artery. However, it was demonstrated, after the internal carotid was opened and the silastic balls introduced, that with the decrease of pressure in the internal carotid such a strong reversal of current occurred that some of the introduced spheres could no longer be transported upward. The operation was therefore limited to the embolization of the internal carotid artery using the spence spheres. Only one ball reached the sack of the aneurysm. Three months later embolization was carried out starting from the vertebral artery, whereby 3 of the 5 silastic balls introduced moved into the aneurysm of the cavernous sinus. Immediately after the operation a pulsating murmur was present which, however, now one year after the operation has disappeared completely. The sinus cavernosus fistula could not be observed.

WÜLLENWEBER: I want to present a case of a huge biparietal angioma which I embolized with 50 - 60 spheres. On the intra-operative angiogram they were nicely lined up in the feeding vessels. The patient awoke, half an hour later and showed decerebration rigidity with a dilated pupil on the side of embolization. On immediate decompression we found extreme edema which was hardly manageable, and the patient died 2 days later. Dr. Luessenhop and Dr. Tzonos have reported only good results. Are there other colleagues who can report a different outcome? My question is addressed to the speakers on artificial embolization.

ERBSLÖH: You must expect that in cases with arteriovenous malformations some emboli go through the shunt into the venous system and cause pulmonary embolism or infarction. How often do you see this complication, or must you expect this complication?

TZONOS: We have embolized 14 patients, 2 of them had increased neurological deficits, but there has been no death so far. We saw only a few pulmonary emboli which I think are of no functional importance.

LUESSENHOP: I have described the complications in other publications, so I did not in this brief presentation elaborate on them. One patient very early in our experience was killed by the procedure. This was a technical mistake. The patient was being embolized via the basilar system, and after some 30 or 40 emboli had gone to the malformation, we became too enthusiastic, and finally they stopped at the bifurcation of the basilar artery. That was an experience that has never happened again. 6 patients in the last 5 or 8 years have had transient but not very serious deficits. I cannot say there is a rule that you can lay down to tell you when to stop embolizing. It is almost like an art. You just have to learn by experience, and if the emboli start to stop proximal to the lesion, you should stop the procedure. Complications of that nature are not important once you have learned the technique. Passage of emboli to the lungs occurs in rare lesions, which have a direct large artery to large vein communication, like in certain malformations to the great vein of Galen. We also had one patient very early in our experience where a great number of emboli passed through immediately or over the next few days. About 40 emboli measuring 3 - 4 mm did pass into the pulmonary circulation. The experts tell me this is nothing to worry about. If you operate this way on very large lesions you should keep careful count every time. You might loose one or two emboli to the lungs, but I think that this is not of any importance. In one case, which was ideal for embolization, the emboli kept going through, and I could not get them to stop in the malformation. So I put a suture on the embolus and held it there with a suture until it stopped, and then I could put others behind it. By this technique I was able to obliterate the lesion. I have never seen edema or a big infarct causing a patient's death.

SANO: When we were using spherical emboli, two patients died, just exactly in the same manner as Dr. Wüllenweber described, because spherical emboli lodged in the main trunk and caused brain edema several hours later. That is why we stopped using spherical emboli. Since we started to use phycon i.e. liquid plastic, we have never seen such a complication. The main trunk is not embolized by liquid plastic. If the arteriovenous shunt is very large, it may be possible that even phycon can pass into the channel, but so far we have not seen this happen.

SEEGER: A short comment on Dr. Wüllenweber's case. I think that the rarity of complications does not depend on the technique itself, but it has more to do with the indications. In our series we had angiomas with many collaterals, and even if the Sylvian artery became occluded, nothing happened. In another case you may have a catastrophe. Well-developed nets of collaterals can prevent it. I would like to ask Dr. Djindjian if he has used gelfoam embolization for internal carotid artery angiomas and what the difficulties or the advantages are.

DJINDJIAN: My experience with embolization of the internal carotid territory is very small. I had two cases, and both of them developed hemiplegia. Therefore I stopped doing it. One of the patients fortunately recovered after several months.

FEINDEL (to LUESSENHOP): Is there any possibility of getting anterior cerebral embolization with cross compression?

LUESSENHOP: The anterior cerebral artery is a big problem, and if the Sylvian artery and anterior cerebral artery are of the same diameter and the angle is not changed, I think the ratio in our experience is about ten to one. You can get a certain number of emboli to go up the anterior cerebral. You noticed those very large malformations I showed - they were mainly in the anterior cerebral territory and there was no problem because the anterior cerebral then becomes the normal anatomical continuation of the internal carotid artery. We have used contralateral compression, but I think you have to be careful when you use it, because you can draw the emboli all the way across into the opposite side. So we have used it very sparingly, but I think that is something to consider. I might make another comment about the edema leading to fatalities. I wonder if this could be related to the amount of contrast media that was used, and the amount of saline used for irrigation during the procedure.

SCHÜRMANN: Besides very large angiomas, are there other indications for the embolization method? What kind and size of emboli do you use?

LUESSENHOP: The primary indication is of course that it cannot be excised. The second would be that anatomically it is suitable. The third would be that the lesion is producing symptoms over and above seizures. The most important thing, however, is that it must be anatomically suitable for embolization. I think it is preferable to have many smaller emboli in the lesion than fewer larger ones slightly proximal to the lesion. We start with the smallest emboli that seem to be safe, but never as small as 1 mm in the internal carotid. The smallest we have ever used in the internal carotid has been 2.5 mm, the largest one being 6 mm. But I would try to get many smaller ones into the lesion first, and near the end one or two slightly larger ones, which will stop proximally. Then they will begin to line up in the feeding arteries. If there are several feeding arteries of different diameter, as Dr. Sano has pointed out, they will all tend to go to the bigger one first, but near the end, as this becomes obliterated, some will begin to enter other smaller arteries, and we keep going very carefully, one at a time, until finally they will go into that other artery. The future of this method lies with what Dr. Djindjian has done and what Dr. Sano has done. We have remained stationary for 14 years, because I did not want to keep changing everything, but I think there is still a long way to go with embolization, and it will be better and even conceivable that someday the big lesions will be completely wiped out.

BRAUN: Dr. Tzonos said that he has had to sacrifice the vertebral or sometimes even the carotid artery after embolization. Do you have to do this with your technique, too?

LUESSENHOP: There were probably some cases where I ligated the internal carotid artery at the end, but not recently. As far as the external carotid, our approach has been the opposite extreme from Dr. Djindjian. We started with embolization via the external carotid, because many of the lesions were supplied by this vessel as well as by the internal carotid early in our experience. So at the end of the procedure we would simply embolize the external carotid artery. After inserting the emboli, we would ligate the external carotid artery. As time passed, we became aware of the other potentialities of the external carotid artery, and we continued in that fashion. I feel the collateral in the external carotid system is so great that the goal of this treatment is to take as much as you possibly can, particularly for large angiomas on the face. We have been very radical in embolizing via the external system and have been most interested in what are the potential complications. We always end the procedure by ligating the external carotid artery, sometimes sparing the superior thyroid and sometimes ligating that as well. We have also done bilateral external carotid ligation, but we never had the occasion to ligate the vertebral artery.

BURNIE: I think it is time to turn this problem over to the physical chemists. They must discover a substance which is soft and pliable when it is cool, and which becomes hard when it is warm. It has to seek the area of greatest flow unerringly. It has to be attracted to and attached to the arterial wall just before it reaches the capillary phase or the venous phase. It has to enlarge slightly when it sticks. It has to be able to be applied directly or through a catheter inserted by any route. And it has to give off a very mild toxic substance that either coagulates or scleroses the vessels just beyond.

PIA: Thank you, Dr. Burnie. I suppose that some of your ideas have been realized already. I would like to ask Dr. Sano to summarize his experience.

SANO: First of all by the present technique all those huge arteriovenous angiomas in the region of M 4 are suitable for treatment and malformations in the region of anterior cerebral artery are unsuitable. Yesterday we heard Dr. Tzonos telling us that they are using fine silicon catheters which can be inserted in any artery of the brain. If this is correct, maybe in the future even those arteriovenous malformations supplied by the anterior or posterior cerebral arteries can be embolized.

PIA (to DJINDJIAN): What do you think will be the future of this embolization technique for angiomas supplied by the internal carotid artery?

DJINDJIAN: The future for me is to try to carry out super-selective arteriography of the Sylvian artery and partial embolization.

Fig. 1 a and b. a) Arteriovenous aneuryms (sinus cavernosus) of the ▶ right internal carotid artery and basilar artery. b) a - p. projection. (Discussion on Chapter VII, HEMMER)

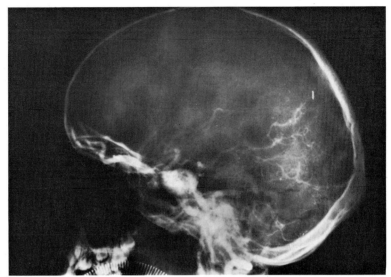

a)

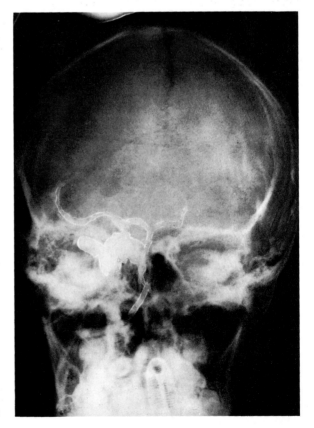

b)

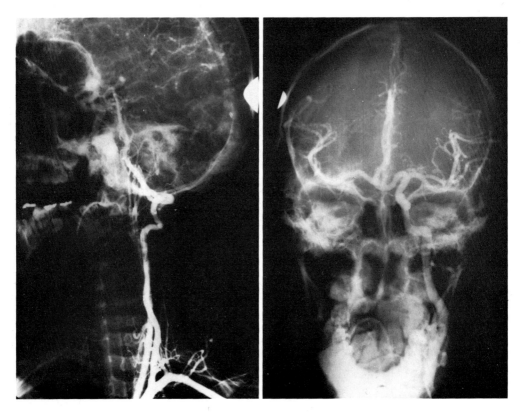

Fig. 2   Fig. 3

Fig. 2. Shows, that the aneurysm is thrombosed, the basilar artery is wholly preserved (supratentorial vessels by simultaneous filling of the left carotid artery).(Discussion on Chapter VII, HEMMER)

Fig. 3. Filling of the carotid artery from the opposite side with complete collateral circulation (a-p). (Discussion on Chapter VII, HEMMER)

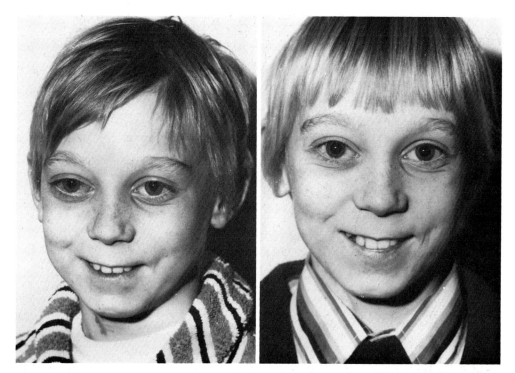

Fig. 4   Fig. 5

Fig. 4. Before embolization, light exophthalmus, noteworthy the vascularisation. (Discussion on Chapter VII, HEMMER)

Fig. 5. One year later. (Discussion on Chapter VII, HEMMER)

Chapter VIII

Radiotherapy

Radiotherapy of Cerebral Angiomas. With a note on some problems in Diagnosis

R. T. JOHNSON

Introduction

Cerebral angiomas have been treated sporadically by various forms of radiotherapy for a considerable time (1). Although clinical improvement occurred in some cases (2), there was no proof that the angioma had been cured and, even if it had, the possibility of spontaneous thrombosis had to be considered. Early cases were exposed at operation as tumour suspects with raised intracranial pressure or as epileptic foci and proved frightening in the days before modern anaesthesia assured a low intracranial pressure with the additional aid of control of the blood pressure. On occasions these large cortical angiomas were submitted to radiotherapy following a, usually necessary, decompression. The treatment was wide field and the maximum effect thought to occur within the first few months. Such a case irradiated in 1944, following sacrifice of the bone flap, presented 16 years later with signs thought to be due to enlargement of the angioma; but an angiogram demonstrated that the right parieto-occipital angioma had disappeared and it was presumed that the symptoms were due to late x-ray necrosis. Refinements in neurological diagnosis and in angiography brought many more angiomas to the rapidly developing skills of neurosurgeons and many more were excised; but still there remained a number considered to be inoperable for one reason or another and many of these patients were submitted to x-ray therapy, although there was no theoretical support for such treatment (3). However, there was no large series on which therapy was accurately controlled and where the results were checked with comprehensive post irradiation angiograms. In fact, angiograms within the first few months of treatment so uniformly demonstrated no change in the angioma that many clinicians considered radiotherapy to be of no avail (4, 5). The realisation that therapy, if effective at all, would be so by producing endarteritis over the sort of time scale that had become recognised as associated with late x-ray necrosis led me to arrange post irradiation angiograms over varying periods - starting at the earliest two years from the last treatment (6).

Material and Methods

One hundred patients either with angiomas considered to be inoperable or who refused operation have been treated over a twenty-year period, initially by Professor Ralston Paterson and later by Professor Eric Easson and his staff at the Radium Institute, Manchester. Basically the patient receives 4,000 to 5,000 rads (depending on the size of the lesion) over a three-week period by megavoltage irradiation beam directed accurately to the centre of the angioma, so that the feeding vessels and draining veins escape the large dosage. This study is continuing and so far detailed examinations have been made on twenty patients by serial angiography at intervals ranging from two to twenty years. There have been 12 angiomas in the posterior cerebral territory (Fig. 1); six have been excised and six treated by irradiation and all have been cured without additional morbidity; it should be noted that some of these angiomas were more anteriorly placed within the thalamus and were not amenable to surgery. There have been a few striking results in posterior fossa angiomas (Fig. 2), but large angiomas in the cerebral cortex have been disappointing (Fig. 3). This was to be expected as the area to be irradiated is much larger and hence the effective dose much lower. To assess changes accurately, comparable angiograms must be carefully selected from a rapid serial run and the angiography must be comprehensive. It is problematical whether irradiation is desirable prior to excision; although it may well reduce the size, the vessels may become arterio-sclerotic and calcified during the long interval; furthermore, vital adjacent irradiated brain may become more vulnerable to the manipulations (anaesthetic and operative) of a surgical procedure. There would seem to be sound reasons for treating all angiomas: many bleed repeatedly (4); some, having caused little disability for a life-time, bleed fatally without warning. Headaches, raised intracranial pressure, loud bruits and fits may be problems and some angiomas increase in size and produce progressive neurological damage: a young engineer with a large left temporal angioma suffered from repeated epileptic attacks and progressive dysphasia (Fig. 4). It is interesting that the technetium scan was positive in his case: actually it has proved a disappointment as a means of monitoring the effects of irradiation; it has been observed to become temporarily positive in cases where serial angiograms have shown no changes, presumably due to transient ischaemia in the surrounding cortex. Some cases are, of course, immediately fatal; others have sustained fatal damage but linger for days or weeks with perplexing signs. It is important to recognise the significance of the draining veins and venous lakes: they become arterialised and thick-walled, but some of the small tributaries from adjacent vital areas of the brain may not share in this and may rupture, causing fatal damage (Fig. 5). Sometimes secondary brainstem haemorrhages render valueless any treatment of the primary lesion, but extensive bleeding into the ventricles may be recoverable. A considerable contribution to the management of the acute case has been made by the introduction of transverse axial tomography by E. M. I. Limited. A patient was admitted to a mental hospital in an acute confused state and, having no localising signs, was found to have heavily blood-stained c. s. f. A scan demonstrated the complete pathological process (Fig. 6).

R e s u l t s

Twenty of the 100 cases irradiated during the past 20 years have so far been examined in angiographic detail. Nine have been totally cured (of these 6 were medially placed in the territory of the posterior cerebral artery, 2 were in the posterior fossa and one was a large surface parieto-occipital angioma); 5 have improved and 5 have shown no change, and in one the angioma is larger (of these all have been large and in the cerebral hemisphere). It is significant that the six medially placed angiomas of medium size have all been cured by irradiation and that the large cortical angiomas have shown little change. The figures are not valid, as the series is as yet incomplete.

Diagnostic Problems

It seems clear that the small or medium sized, medially placed angioma responds well to radiotherapy and without recognisable complications, over periods ranging from three to seven years. Detailed angiography (selective, tomographic or stereographic) may demostrate and locate small areas of the large inoperable angioma, which might be cured if these areas were selectively irradiated. LEXSELL (7) has developed a Gamma unit for irradiating to destruction small areas in the brain stereotactically and has had some success with selective thrombosis of vessels in massive angiomas (8); an interesting and important observation, considering how ineffective the operation of multiple clipping of the main supplying vessels has proved to be. It might be that the aneurysmal formations in large angiomas, which are frequently the site of haemorrhage - especially into the ventricles (4)- could be selectively treated. Small angiomas may not show on routine angiography and their presence is only revealed by a filling defect in the ventricular pattern produced by the venous 'aneurysms' associated with them (Fig. 7). An identical case has since been successfully diagnosed and treated by ventriculo-cisternostomy and radiotherapy. More striking are the enormous venous lakes with the dural angiomas: small insignificant angiomas supplied by meningeal arteries and sometimes only filled on selective angiography. In two recent cases the venous aneurysm was confined to the posterior fossa and filled only from one carotid. Surgery is difficult, so irradiation focused on the areas of dural supply might be the best mode of treatment.

Acknowledgements

To Miss DOROTHY DAVISON, former medical artist, University of Manchester, for Figs. 5, 7; to Dr. IAN ISHERWOOD of the Department of Neuro-Radiology, Manchester Royal Infirmary, for the E. M. I. scans (Fig. 6) and the angiograms; and to Dr. R. G. W. OLLERENSHAW of the Department of Medical Illustration, University of Manchester, for the photographs.

Summary

A preliminary report is presented on the results of irradiating inoperable cerebral angiomas. Of the twenty cases fully documented 45 per cent have been cured, 25 per cent improved and 25 per cent not changed, and success has been almost, but not totally, related to size. Refinements in diagnosis may enable selective therapy to improve the results in the larger angiomas.

References

1. CUSHING, H., BAILEY, P.: "Tumours arising from the blood vessels of the brain", Springfield, Ill.: Thomas 1928.

2. POTTER, J. M.: "Angiomatous Malformations of the Brain: their nature and prognosis", Ann. Roy. Col. Surgeons of England 16, 227-243 (1955).

3. KRENCHEL, N. J.: "Intracranial Racemose Angiomas: A Clinical Study", p. 102, 103, Aarhus: Universitetsforlaget 1961.

4. JEFFERSON, G.: "Les hemorrhagies sous-arachnoidiennes par angiomes et aneurysmes chez le jeune", Rev. Neurol. 80, 413-432 (1948).

5. OLIVECRONA, H., LADENHEIM, J.: "Congenital arterio-venous aneurysms of the carotid and vertebral systems". Springer: Berlin 1957.

6. JOHNSON, R. T.: "Surgery of Cerebral Haemorrhage", Lord Brain and Marcia Wilkinson (eds.): Recent Advances in Neurology, p. 124-126. London: Churchill 1969.

7. LEXSELL, L.: "Cerebral Radiosurgery", Gammathalamotomy in two cases of intractable pain, Acta Chir. Scand. 134, 585 (1968).

8. LEXSELL, L.: "Personal Communication" (1973).

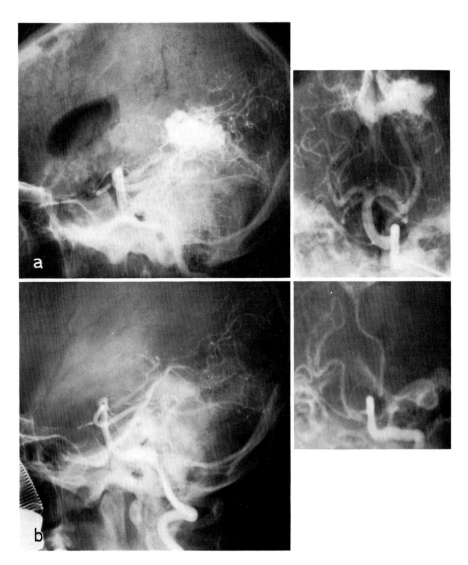

Fig. 1 a and b. Posterior cerebral angioma: vertebral angiogram, lateral and anterior-posterior projections: a) pre-radiotherapy; b) six years post radiotherapy. This angioma is posterior to the thalamus and could have been excised

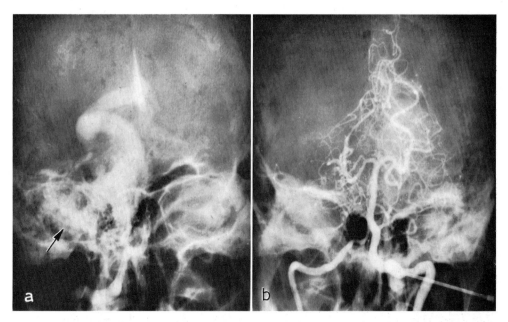

Fig. 2 a and b. Posterior fossa angioma: vertebral angiograms: a) pre-radiotherapy - angioma (↗) on left side with rapid shunt into large venous channel; b) three years post radiotherapy - both vertebral arteries are filled, there is no shunt and probably no angiomatous vessels

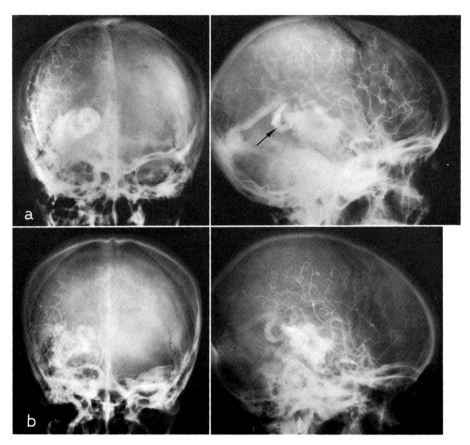

Fig. 3 a and b. Temporal angioma: right carotid angiograms (anterior-
posterior and lateral: a) pre-radiotherapy - large, deeply placed angioma draining through the great cerebral vein (↗) into the straight
sinus; b) four years post radiotherapy - angioma still large, but some
slight reduction in size and shunt. Persistent severe headaches and
repeated subarachnoid haemorrhages necessitated excision of the angioma, which was successfully completed in stages 12 years later

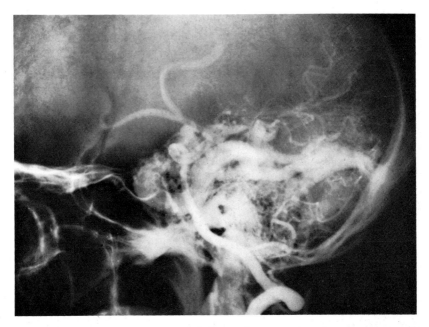

Fig. 4. Left temporal angioma: vertebral angiogram showing enormous
dilatation of the draining veins; total excision for disabling dysphasia resulted in considerable improvement

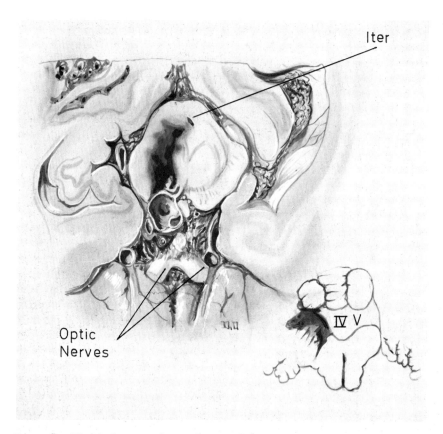

Fig. 5. Right temporal angioma: death from haemorrhage into the mid-brain and floor of the fourth ventricle. Angioma almost identical to that in Fig. 4. Section of mid-brain from below showing dilated vein in the interpeduncular fossa, a tributary of which had ruptured into the peduncle and thence down into the right side of the floor of the 4th ventricle (inset). The patient survived for some weeks with a left hemiplegia, responding only to pain

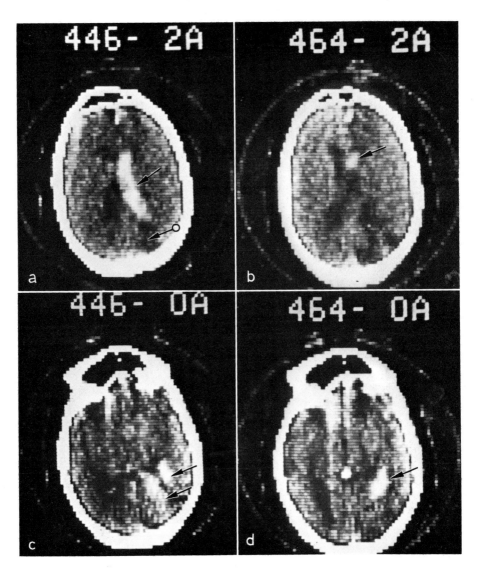

Fig. 6 a – d. E.M.I. scan: polaroid prints of the transverse axial to-
mograms: a) the right lateral ventricle is full of blood clot (↙) and
posterior to it is an area representing angioma and oedematous brain
tissue (↙); b) the same section a few days later and following a burr
hole and aspiration of the ventricle - residual clot in the anterior
horn (↙); c) a lower section through the frontal sinuses (above) showing clots in the trigone and temporal horn on the right (↙↙); d) after
aspiration of residual clot in the temporal horn (↙). The angioma was
later excised from the ventricular wall

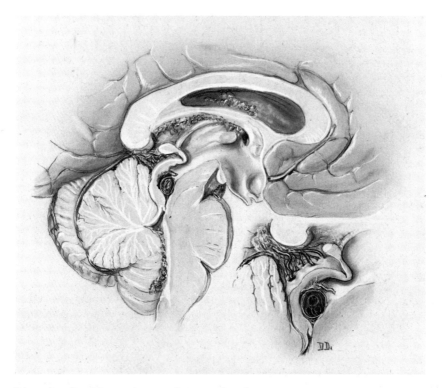

Fig. 7. Small angioma of tectal plate; saggital section showing medial aspect of left side of brain; sudden death caused by total obstruction of iter. The angioma is represented solely by the fine arterial filaments perforating the tectal plate and the solitary dilated venous channel lying in the iter which thrombosed (inset)

Discussion on Chapter VIII

PIA: All of us learned that OLIVECRONA absolutely turned down radio-therapy for a-v angiomas. We know, however, about successful cases, last presented by Dr. Potter in a collective review. So there is no doubt that it can be effective where the size, shape, and extent of the shunt may have a decisive effect.

LUESSENHOP (to JOHNSON): Do you have the impression that perhaps the danger of hemorrhage is increased during the period of X-ray therapy because of necrosis of the vessels involved?

JOHNSON: I do not really think so. One case who died really had not had any effective X-ray therapy. The others have been two patients who had odd symptoms at the end of a period of time and this was the stage where we found that the angioma had been cured. It might be that they had an active time of thrombosis.

FEINDEL: I would just like to suggest that the very simple bilateral or even unilateral intravenous isotope study, using the old-fashioned detector which gives you a simple transient time, can be quite useful in following up some of these patients. It is not valid for blood flow, but it does give you an interesting comparison, and we have used that because it is a very simple thing to do. It is even·simpler than an-giography.

JOHNSON: But could you be absolutely sure that the angioma was cured?

FEINDEL: No. But if you do a preoperative set of curves under the same conditions and follow them along, you do have a comparative basis. So it is of some value if you can get the patient to cooperate to have an arteriogram.

Chapter IX
The Natural History

Conservative Management of Inoperable Arteriovenous Malformations

G. E. PERRET

It is agreed by most authors dealing with Arteriovenous Malformations (AVM) that most bleeding lesions with intraparenchymal hematoma and recurring hemorrhages producing increasing neurologic deficit should be treated surgically (1, 2). However, it is obviously not advisable to operate if the lesion cannot be completely excised, and if the patient's condition is worsened by the procedure (3, 4, 5). The operative risk is definitely increased by the location and extent of the malformation. The age of the patient, his general condition, the presence of other diseases, and certain social factors should also be considered in evaluating the operative risk and a possible postoperative neurologic deficit (1, 6). A relatively asymptomatic lesion may make a surgical approach inadvisable when considering the possible risks involved.

The Cooperative Study (6) has shown that death from an aneurysm rupture is more common (36% of subarachnoid hemorrhage (SAH) than death from a bleeding AVM (2% SAH). However, 90% of the patients dying within 72 hours of a SAH had an intracranial, mostly intracerebral hematoma. When a hemorrhage is due to AVM, 24% of death occurred within 24 hours, 27% within 48 hours. A large portion of death from AVMs occurs earlier than from aneurysm, but after the third week, the proportion of death is much lower than for aneurysms. As shown in my earlier report, the incidence of rebleeding and the incidence of neurologic deficits is greater in inoperable AVMs. However, the survival rate is as good as in other AVMs.

Activities related to onset of hemorrhage is generally the same for AVM as for aneurysms. Hemorrhage occurs during sleep in 36% of the cases, in unspecified circumstances 28%, when lifting or bending 14%, produced by emotional strain 5.9%, defecation 4.1%, coitus 4.1%, coughing 1.3%, urination 1.5%, parturition 0.5%. The only exception is trauma. It is more commonly associated with the onset of SAH from AVM, probably because AVM is more common in young people who are more prone to vigorous activity (4.4% vs 2.8% in aneurysms) (6).

It is very doubtful that changes in daily activities of the patient with AVM would avoid or precipitate recurrent hemorrhages.

Reports on intra- and paraventricular and brain stem AVM successfully treated by surgery are available (2, 5). However, these lesions are still considered inoperable by most neurosurgeons (7, 8, 9).

Incomplete excision or ligation of feeding arteries or ligation of one carotid artery in the neck in an attempt to decrease the blood flow through the AVM has been shown to be useless and may aggrevate the patient's condition by depriving the normal brain of an adequate blood supply (1, 5). Ligation of visible arteries is also useless as other more deeply situated vessels will enlarge to fill the lesion (1).

Palliative therapy consisting of external or tentorial decompression (10) or simple removal of an intracerebral hematoma (9) has occasionally been of benefit to the patient. Increased intracranial pressure secondary to obstructive hydrocephalus produced by intraventricular, midbrain or brain stem AVM may successfully be reduced by various types of shunting procedures (3, 4, 11).

Artificial embolization has been successful in relatively small AVMs fed by primarily the middle cerebral artery (12). However, not all vessels supplying a lesion are equally enlarged. Emboli may obstruct some but not others (4). This method is probably of little help in AVMs fed by 2, 3 or 4 main arterial trunks as is frequently encountered in the paraventricular region. Cryotherapy and radio frequency thrombosis of the AVMs are new methods impossible to fully evaluate at the present time.

Deep roentgen irradiation has been used by many (13). Its effectiveness is minimal and may have a damaging effect on the surrounding brain tissue (4, 14, 15).

Convulsive seizures are rarely uncontrollable. They are best treated symptomatically with anticonvulsants. Most authors agree that convulsions alone are not an indication for surgical treatment of the AVM. The incidence of convulsions may be unchanged if not increased by surgical treatment (5, 16).

From our clinical experience, it appears that anti-edema agents, such as mannitol, glycerol, urea and dexamethasone and fluid restriction benefit the patient after a hemorrhage. Clinical and experimental data suggest that antifibrinolytic agents, such as epsilonaminocaproic acid and tranexamic acid decrease the rate of recurrent hemorrhage from an aneurysm and may perhaps prevent early recurrent bleeding from an AVM.

S u m m a r y

Conservative treatment of inoperable AVMs is essentially symptomatic and is confined to the control of convulsive seizures, hydrocephalus & cerebral edema.

R e f e r e n c e s

1. FRENCH, L. A., STORY, J. L.: Cerebrovascular Malformations. Clin. Neurosurg. 11, p. 171-182 (1964).

2. MOODY, R. A., POPPEN, J. L.: Arteriovenous Malformations. J. Neurosurg. 32, 503-511 (1970).

3. KRAYENBÜHL, H.: Discussion on Supratentorial Angiomas. First International Congress of Neurosurgery, p.263-267. Brussels (1957).

4. FRENCH, L. A., CHOU, S. N.: Conventional Methods of Treating Intracranial Arteriovenous Malformations. Prog. Neurol. Surg. 3, p. 274-319. Basel: Karger & Chicago: Year Book (1969).

5. AMACHER, A. L., ALCOCK, J. M., DRAKE, C. G.: Cerebral Angiomas; The Sequelae of Surgical Treatment. J. Neurosurg. 37, 571-575 (1972).

6. LOCKSLEY, H. B.: Natural History of Subarachnoid Hemorrhage, Intracranial Aneurysms & Arteriovenous Malformations. In: Sahs, A.L., Perret, G. E., Locksley, H. B., Nishioka, H. (eds.): Intracranial Aneurysms and Subarachnoid Hemorrhage; A Cooperative Study. Philadelphia & Toronto: J. B. Lippincott Co. 1969.

7. GILLINGHAM, J.: Arteriovenous Malformations of the Head. Edinb. Med. Journ. 60, 305-319 (1953).

8. PATERSON, J. H., MCKISSOCK, W.: A clinical Survey of Intracranial Angiomas with Special Reference to Their Mode of Progression & Surgical Treatment. Brain. 79, 233-266 (1956).

9. MCKISSOCK, W., HANKINSON, J.: The Surgical Treatment of Supratentorial Angiomas. First International Congress of Neurosurgery, p. 223-228. Brussels (1957).

10. LOGUE, V., MONCKTON, G.: Posterior Fossa Angiomas. Brain 77, 252-273 (1954).

11. KELLY, D. L., ALEXANDER, E., DAVUS, C. H., MAYNARD, D. C.: Intracranial Arteriovenous Malformations. Clinical Review & Evaluation of Brain Scans. J. Neurosurg. 31, 422-428 (1969).

12. LUESSENHOP, A. J.: Artificial Embolization for Cerebral Arteriovenous Malformations. Progr. Neurol. Surg. 3, p. 320-362. Basel: Karger & Chicago: Year Book (1969).

13. POTTER, J. M.: Angiomatous Malformations of the Brain; Their Nature & Prognosis. Ann. Roy. Coll. Surg. Engl. 16, 227-242 (1955).

14. OLIVECRONA, H., LADENHEIM, J.: Arteriovenous Aneurysms of the Carotid and Vertebral Arterial Systems, IV, 91 p. Berlin: Springer-Verlag (1957).

15. POOL, J. J.: Treatment of Arteriovenous Malformations of the Cerebral Hemispheres. J. Neurosurg. 19, 136-141 (1962).

16. FORSTER, D. M. C., STEINER, L., HAKANSON, S.: Arteriovenous Malformations of the Brain; A Long-Term Clinical Study. J. Neurosurg. 37, 562-570 (1972).

Conservative Treatment of Cerebral Arteriovenous Angiomas

W. WALTER

The concept of conservative treatment of arteriovenous angiomas of the brain must be questioned right from the start, since there is no active treatment apart from surgery. Basically, refusing operation means hoping for a more or less favorable clinical course. X-ray treatment which was often applied formerly is no longer thought of today. Follow-up studies of patients from TÖNNIS' case material, who had undergone x-ray therapy indicated that this treatment does not affect the clinical course in the least. Sometimes, x-ray treatment even led to deterioration. According to our pathophysiological concepts about the hemodynamic effects of arteriovenous angiomas on the circulation of adjacent brain tissue, as well as on the cerebral circulation as a whole, the effects of x-ray therapy are likely to be damaging. Thus, recommendations for "conservative treatment" mean only a quiet way of life to avoid recurrent hemorrhages and antiepileptic medication to minimize the risk of seizures.

However, experience shows that recurrent hemorrhages occur even in patients who live very quietly (furthermore, the patient often does not or cannot lead a quiet life). As far as antiepileptic therapy is concerned, we are under the impression that seizures due to angiomas are more difficult to treat than epileptic seizures from other causes. This is supported by the fact that the treatment drug used was frequently changed in over 50% of the patients with seizures. Therefore the decision to undertake conservative treatment can be made only after due considerations by the physician and his patient, who must weigh the risk of the operation against the future clinical course without operation. Subjective elements play a considerable role here both in the advice of surgeons (among whom the readiness to take a risk is not evenly distributed) and in the personality of the patient. The surgeon advising the patient must be guided not only by his own experience and the reported good and bad results of operations but he must also consider the possible and calculable dangers of so-called conservative treatment.

There are 3 criteria for the evaluation of this question:

1. Is the chronic limitation of the cerebral circulation likely to increase through the arteriovenous shunt? In other words, are increasing psychological changes in the sense of mental deterioration or neurological deficits to be expected?

2. How great is the danger of a new hemorrhage both with regard to its incidence and its possible lethal consequences?

3. Can the occurrence of epileptic seizures with all their consequences
   (such as psychological deterioration) be influenced? In other words,
   will the tendency progress, remain stationary, undergo improvement
   or even cease after anticonvulsive treatment?

The first question, whether circulatory disturbance increases has been
repeatedly answered by publications reporting enlargement of the angioma on control angiography. Although there is no autochtonous growth
as in tumors, observation does show that there is an enlargement of
the arteriovenous shunt with a corresponding change in hemodynamic re-
lationships within the brain (Figs. 1a, 1b, 2a, 2b). The traumatic arteriovenous carotid-cavernous fistula serves as a good model for these
changes since the exact time at which the fistula occurred is known
and the interval till the performance of the angiogramm easily determined.

As the diagrams show (Figs. 3, 4, 6a, 6b) the circulation becomes worse,
the longer the shunt remains. Analogous to the findings of RAU, HEBERER
and EBERLEIN in the case of traumatic arteriovenous fistulae involving
large blood vessels in the body, certain changes occur especially in
the venous side of the circulation. The drop in arterial pressure near
the fistula with a simultaneous rise in venous pressure leads to venous
hypertension. The pictures show that the changes in the venous side
with the formation of numerous hypertrophic draining veins, increase
the longer the fistula remains. This can lead to such grotesque situations that ultimately the cerebral circulation finally consists only
of large varicosities in which the contrast medium disappears. Similar changes of a lesser degree are certainly to be expected in the case
of arteriovenous angiomas as well. The probability that such changes
will occur becomes greater if the original angioma is already very
large. The mental changes in patients with angiomata were studied in
our own case material as well as that of LANGE-COSACK and were attributed to this mechanism.

The second question, i.e. the question of recurrent hemorrhage, is certainly not as important here as in the case of saccular aneurysms. The
general impression is that these hemorrhages are not so serious, and
that they do not recur so frequently. The fact that these hemorrhages
run a more benign course is confirmed by the experience that 50% of
the bleeds in our patient material were not recognized during childhood or young adulthood because they run a relatively minor and undra-
matic course (Fig. 5).

The epileptic seizures - 40 - 50 % of the patients have seizures alone
- are the predominant symptom if the angioma is located in the centro-
parietal region and are much rarer if the angioma is situated elsewhere.
Jacksonian seizures and generalized seizures occur with equal frequency. There are two observations which are typical for seizures due to
arteriovenous angiomas over the course of several years:

a) Postparoxysmal pareses or aphasic disturbances, regardless of whether they are transient or permanent, are much more common than with
   seizures due to other causes. This probably also leads to increasing seizure activity over the course of years and new neurological
   deficits which render the patient unable to work.

b) The incidence of seizure activity is very variable. We know of patients with seizures occuring only at great intervals and then again
   those who suffer from series of them. The common experience is that
   anticonvulsant treatment generally has little success and is difficult to manage.

A survey of the histories of 50 non-operated patients show that although approximately 60% have a more or less downhill course, no less than 40% had no difficulties, and, in particular, no complaints (Fig. 7). The majority of these had smaller angiomas which were not operated upon because either the angiomas were inoperable because of their position or the patients refused the operation. Although total removal should be attempted, these observations with non-operated patients cannot be overlooked. Again and again we will find ourselves in the situation of having to advise for or against operation when the angioma is in a particularly dangerous location. Among these patients, some of whom have lived for years with an angioma, there are certainly some in whom the effort to perform total removal would have led to death or severe neurological deficit. We can only hope that the methods discussed here for treating angiomas previously considered inoperable will simplify the considerations and decision regarding the indications for operation.

R e f e r e n c e s

1. HEBERER, G., RAU, G., EBERLEIN, H. J.: Langenbecks Arch. klin. Chir. 299, 254, (1962).

2. TÖNNIS, W., WALTER, W.: Warum Totalexstirpation der intracraniellen arteriovenösen Angiome? Zu: Leistung und Ergebnisse der neuzeitl. Chirurgie. Stuttgart: Thieme 1958.

3. TÖNNIS, W., SCHIEFER, W.: Zirkulationsstörungen des Gehirns im Serienangiogramm. Berlin: Springer 1959.

4. TÖNNIS, W., WALTER, W., FRIEDMANN, G.: Störungen der Hirndurchblutung bei arteriovenösen Angiomen des Gehirns. Arch. Kreisll.-Forsch. 31, 135 (1959).

5. TÖNNIS, W., WALTER, W.: Die Indikation zur Totalexstirpation der intracraniellen arteriovenösen Angiome. Wtsch. 2. Nervenheilk. 186, 279 (1964).

6. TÖNNIS, W., WALTER, W., BROCK, M.: Die Totalexstirpation intracerebraler arteriovenöser Angiome bei Lokalisation im funktionell wichtigen Hirnrealen. Betr. Neurochir., Heft 11. Leipzig: Barth 1966.

7. WALTER, W.: Klinik, Diagnostik und oz. Behandl. der intracran. Gefäßmißbildung und nicht-traumat. Blutungen. Habilitationsschrift Köln 1965.

8. WALTER, W., BISCHOF, W.: Die Durchblutungsstörung des Gehirns bei sinus-cavernosus Aneurysmen. Zbl. f. Neurochir. 27 H. 3, 139-155 (1966).

9. WALTER, W.: Neurologische Komplikationen nach Exstirpation arteriovenöser Angiome im funktionell wichtigen Hirnrealen. Dtsch. Kongreß für Neurochirurgie Bad Dürkheim 1966 (Kongreßband).

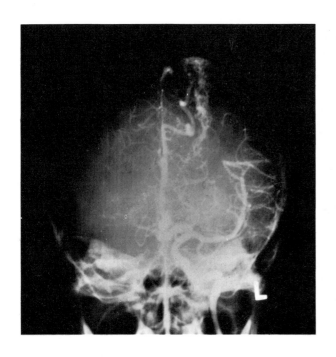

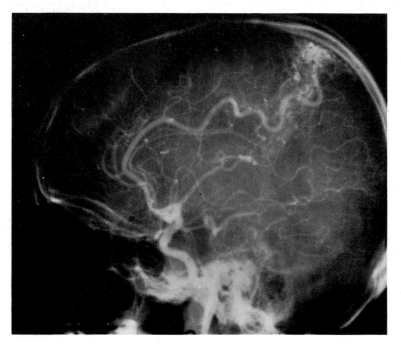

Fig. 1 a and b. Arteriovenous angioma, relatively small and circumscribed

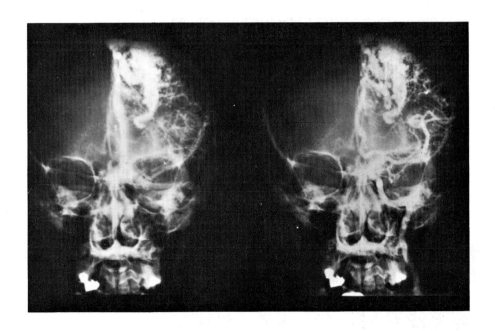

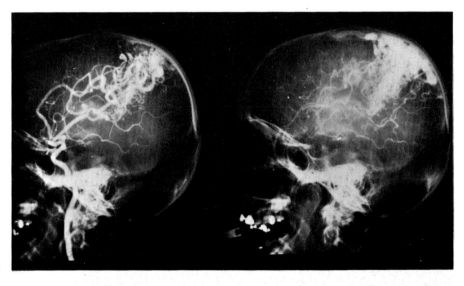

Fig. 2 a and b. Repeat angiogram of the same patient 9 years later. Distinct enlargement of the angioma with increased number and size of draining veins

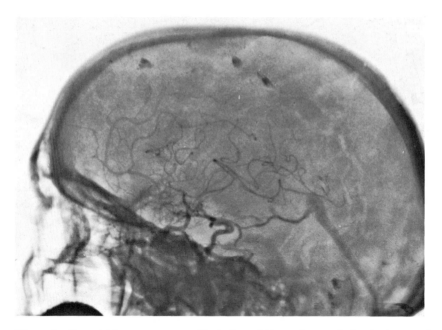

Fig. 3. Carotid-cavernous fistula with enlarged draining veins after 6 months without treatment

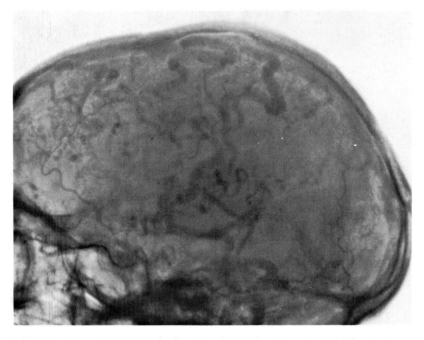

Fig. 4. Carotid-cavernous fistula untreated for 2 years. Marked formation of numerous enlarged draining veins

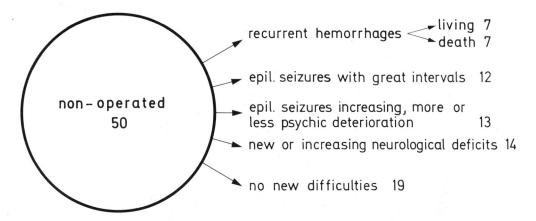

recurrent hemorrhages ⟨ living 7 / death 7

epil. seizures with great intervals 12

epil. seizures increasing, more or less psychic deterioration 13

new or increasing neurological deficits 14

no new difficulties 19

non-operated 50

Fig. 5. Recurrent hemorrhage in cases of angiomata

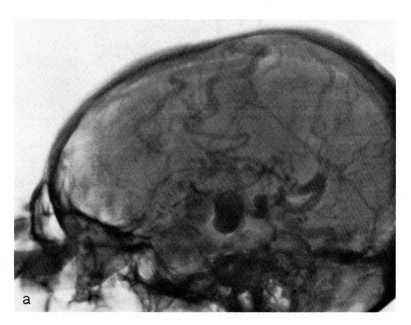

Fig. 6 a. Massive "varicosity" of a carotid-cavernous fistula untreated for 18 years

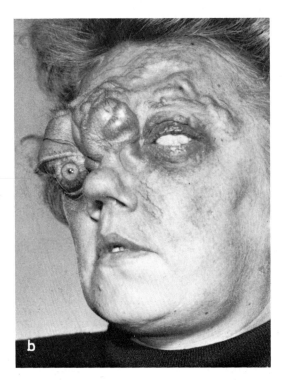

Fig. 6 b. Same patient (angiogram Fig. 6 a) untreated carotid-cavernous fistula for 18 years

Intervals of recurrent hemorrhages

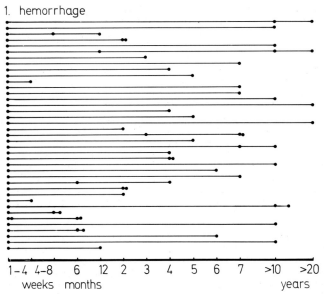

Fig. 7. Histories of unoperated angiomas over a period of 2 - 15 years

Summary and Conclusions

This meeting dealt almost exclusively with practical problems encountered in the management of inoperable intracerebral angiomas. We have defined an inoperable angioma as a malformation, which cannot be totally excised or occluded by classical neurosurgical techniques without producing severe neurological deficits, either because it is located in the central regions of the brain or because it involves functionally and vitally important areas. We did not expect to find any solutions, and it would be wrong to lay down any cast-iron principles of management, particularly as far as the choice of operative treatment and the surgical technique is concerned. This is simply due to the fact that many of the recently developed techniques reflect the diverse experiences of individual surgeons, and the number of patients subjected to treatment with newly developed techniques is still small. Personal experience, technical skill, and other individual factors will continue to determine to a great extent the decision of whether the malformation is "operable" or not.

As far as epidemiology is concerned, it appears that approximately one fourth to one third of cerebral arteriovenous malformations seen either by the clinician or pathologist will come into the category of inoperable angioma.

Thanks to the Cooperative Study and to other reports presented here, we obtained a well documented and unbiased picture of the natural history of cerebral arteriovenous malformations. Before the surgical correction of a malformation is attempted, such factors as the risk and possible severity of the hemorrhage, the presence of a cerebral steal, the possibility of increasing mental and neurological deficits; the presence or the risk of epilepsy and the possibility of its control, have to be analysed and weighed against the risk of all the types of treatment available today. The reports presented here enable one to calculate that risk in percentages, but as PERRET said, for the individual patient the behaviour of the arteriovenous malformation is unpredictable, and there are no factors that point to a particularly bad or good prognosis.

As far as diagnosis is concerned, recent years have brought a considerable refinement of angiographic techniques, including angiocinematography and magnification angiography. It appears that intraoperative angiography should become routine in the surgery of deep-seated angiomas. Pre- and intraoperative measurement of the cerebral circulation time and fluorescin angiography as developed by FEINDEL and his group are of considerable importance in establishing the presence of a cerebral steal, about which angiography alone gives only limited information. These techniques also help in lessening the risk of increased postoperative neurological deficit. Apart from contributing to our understanding of the cerebral steal syndrome, another fact, which makes these investigations so valuable, is that as has been demonstrated, this combined technique is applicable in practice in the operating theatre.

The advantages of the EMI scanner in the diagnosis of intracerebral lesions is already well-known. Its main value, as far as vascular malformations are concerned, is the fact that it makes possible the rapid differentiation between hemorrhage, infarction, and oedema that it can establish the extent of hemorrhage and that it can diagnose bleeding into the ventricle.

Superselective angiography, and its natural sequel superselective embolization, as developed by DJINDJIAN, gave a completely new look to the management of malformations supplied by the external carotid and subclavian system. It seems not to be an exaggeration to say that this technique revolutionizes the diagnosis and treatment of vascular malformations of the head and neck and gives to the neuroradiologist a therapeutic tool. As well as neurosurgeons, it must interest dental surgeons, ENT surgeons, and plastic surgeons. It is only natural that superselective internal carotid angiography and embolization provoked considerable discussion, and the general feeling was that this will be feasible in the not too distant future. However, at this moment it remains in the experimental phase.

Surgery of deep-seated paraventricular angiomas has been facilitated by the use of the microscope and stereotactic localization of the feeding vessels combined with microsurgical clipping.

This last technique decreases the risk of damage to the surrounding tissue in the approach to the malformation.

Operations on cerebellar angiomas provided the latter are not located in the superior vermis, are relatively safe and meet with good results. However, the results on malformations located in the region of the quadrigeminal plate, near the great vein of Galen, or affecting the pons and mesencephalon, seem to indicate that in spite of extremely skilful techniques only partial clipping was possible in more than half the patients upon whom operations were performed.

Patients with intracerebral and intraventricular hematomas caused by hemorrhage from an angioma can be operated upon in the acute phase by a one-stage procedure with subsequent low mortality and morbidity.

Cryosurgery introduced by WALDER has not fulfilled entirely his expectations, but has proved to be a valuable additional method, especially in deep-seated angiomas.

Techniques of embolization introduced by LUESSENHOP 14 years ago, were extensively discussed and became one of the main topics of the workshop. Several modifications of the original technique have been introduced in recent years.

That introduced by SANO, who uses a liquid plastic material, aims at occlusion of the malformation itself, and thus produces embolization more distally than occurs in the technique of LUESSENHOP. This seems to increase the chances of diminishing the shunt present in a malformation with multiple feeders.

280

Embolization has become a widely accepted procedure, particularly for angiomas supplied by feeders from the middle cerebral artery, but it must be remembered that the aim of embolization is to reduce the volume of the malformation in order to diminish the extent of the cerebral steal, the importance of which has been so strongly stressed during the workshop. This does not seem to reduce the risk of further seizures or recurrent hemorrhage as the complete occlusion of the lesion is possible only exceptionally.

The effects of radiotherapy on arteriovenous malformations has been questioned in the past, and this kind of treatment is at present regarded as completely useless. However, the long-term effects of this kind of treatment have been neglected so far and have escaped evaluation.

Yet, if the definition of inoperability of arteriovenous malformation formulated during our meeting is supplemented by a second statement, to which all participants have agreed and which says that the ideal treatment is the complete excision or occlusion of the malformation, partial excision or ligation of feeding vessels being useless, we must conclude that we are still far away from that aim. We felt, however, that considerable steps have been made and new concepts in diagnosis and treatment have been developed and established. There is also good reason to hope that the new therapeutic measures presented here will be further improved in the very near future.

Subject Index

The letters "ff" printed in the subject index mean that the word in question at least appears on the two or even on the four following pages.

A. Wackenheim, J.P. Braun
Angiography of the Mesencephalon
Normal and Pathological Findings
128 figures. XI, 154 pages. 1970
ISBN 3-540-05266-6
Cloth DM 108,—
ISBN 0-387-05266-6
(North America) Cloth US $33.10

**Radiological Exploration
of the Ventricles
and Subarachnoid Space**
By G. Ruggiero, J. Bories, A. Calabrò,
G. Cristi, G. Scialfa, F. Smaltino,
A. Thibaut. With the cooperation
of G. Gianasi, G. Maranghi,
C. Philippart, E. Signorini
90 partly colored figures
(279 separate illustrations)
XIV, 152 pages. 1974
ISBN 3-540-06572-5
Cloth DM 148,—
ISBN 0-387-06572-5
(North America) Cloth US $60.70
Distribution rights for Japan:
Igaku Shoin Ltd., Tokyo

Advances in Neurosurgery

Vol. 1: **Brain Edema**
Pathophysiology and Therapy

Cerebello Pontine Angle Tumors
Diagnosis and Surgery
Editors: K. Schürmann, M. Brock,
H.-J. Reulen, D. Voth
187 figures. XVII, 385 pages. 1973
ISBN 3-540-06486-6
DM 60,—
ISBN 0-387-06486-6
(North America) US $23.10
Distribution rights for Japan:
Nankodo Co. Ltd., Tokyo

L.G. Kempe
Operative Neurosurgery
Distribution rights for Japan:
Nankodo Co. Ltd., Tokyo

Vol. 1: **Cranial, Cerebral, and
Intracranial Vascular Disease**
335 figures, some in color
XIII, 269 pages. 1968
ISBN 3-540-04208-3
Cloth DM 190,—
ISBN 0-387-04208-3
(North America) Cloth US $55.60

Vol. 2: **Posterior Fossa, Spinal Cord,
and Peripheral Nerve Disease**
290 figures, some in color
VIII, 281 pages. 1970
ISBN 3-540-04890-1
Cloth DM 190,—
ISBN 0-387-04890-1
(North America) Cloth US $77.60

Prices are subject to change
without notice

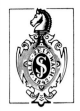

**Springer-Verlag
Berlin
Heidelberg
New York**

Cerebral Circulation and Metabolism
6th International Symposium
Editor: M. Reivich
216 figures. 82 tables
Approx. 530 pages. 1974
In preparation
ISBN 3-540-06645-4
ISBN 0-387-06645-4
(North America)
Distribution rights for Japan:
Nankodo Co. Ltd., Tokyo

Cerebral Circulation and Stroke II
Newer Contributions of the Salzburg
Conference
In preparation

Intracranial Pressure
Experimental and Clinical Aspects
Editors: M. Brock, H. Dietz
142 figures. XVI, 383 pages. 1972
ISBN 3-540-06039-1
Cloth DM 78,—
ISBN 0-387-06039-1
(North America) Cloth US $29.30
Distribution rights for Japan:
Igaku Shoin Ltd., Tokyo

K.J. Zülch
Atlas of Gross
Neurosurgical Pathology
379 figures. VIII, 228 pages. 1975
ISBN 3-540-06480-X
Cloth DM 120,—
ISBN 0-387-06480-X
(North America) Cloth US $49.00
Distribution rights for Japan:
Nankodo Co. Ltd., Tokyo

K.J. Zülch
Atlas of the Histology
of Brain Tumors
Title and text in six languages
(English, German, French, Spanish,
Russian, and Japanese)

100 figures. XVI, 261 pages. 1971
ISBN 3-540-05274-7
Cloth DM 88,—
ISBN 0-387-05274-7
(North America) Cloth US $26.80
Distribution rights for Japan:
Nankodo Co. Ltd., Tokyo

Classification of Brain Tumours
Report of the International Sympo-
sium at Cologne 30 August—1 Sep-
tember, 1961. Sponsored by the
Max-Planck-Gesellschaft, The
Deutsche Forschungsgemeinschaft,
The World Federation of Neurology.
Editors: K.J. Zülch, A.L. Woolf
First Edition 1964 — reprinted 1965.
71 figures. X, 218 pages. 1965
(Acta Neurochirurgica, Supplemen-
tum X).
ISBN 3-211-80712-8
DM 70,—
ISBN 0-387-80712-8
(North America) US $27.00

Prices are subject to change
without notice

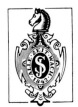

Springer-Verlag
Berlin
Heidelberg
New York